THE COMPLETE GUIDE TO A PLANT-BASED DIET

2 Books in 1:

Guide for Beginners and High Protein Cookbook

Reset and Energize Your Body, Lose Weight, Improve Your Nutrition and Muscle Growth with Delicious Vegetable Recipes. Includes 2 meal plan

Sarah Brown

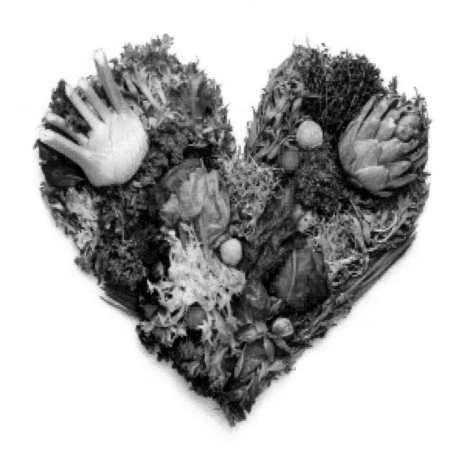

Table of contents:

PLANT-BASED DIET
FOR BEGINNERS

Introduction

In this Book you will also discover why a plant based diet does so many good things for you as well as how to easily implement the delicious recipes in this cookbook into your daily meals. A plant-based diet is a great way to become healthier, happier, more productive and have a lot more energy! Some of the foods included in a plant based diet are vegetables, nuts, seeds, beans, fruits, whole grains and more. Plant-based diets can be vegetarian or vegan, but they may also include certain dairy products and meat if you desire. In fact, vegetarian and vegan diets are only a couple of the many forms of plant-based diets that are popular today.

It is a proven fact that eating less meat and fewer animal-derived foods along with a plant based diet does make most people healthier and helps them to maintain a healthy weight. Plant-based diets are largely successful because they eliminate the use of processed foods that can adversely affect our bodies while fueling the body with natural and healthy foods.

Changing to a plant-based diet can result to be a really important decision you can make to improve your health, your energy, and also prevent different diseases. Science show that you can live longer by eating in a healthy way; you can also help the environment and reduce the risk of getting sick.

This cookbook gives you the opportunity to take care of yourself in a simple, affordable, and delicious way by nourishing your body in a healthy way. Start cooking with these plant-based recipes today as making this change could save your life!

With this cookbook, you will enjoy simple and delicious plant-based diet meals that you will love and eat again and again!

In this book you will find delicious and simple plant-based recipes that will be suitable even for those who only start their Plant Based journey.

Here we go...

Chapter 1: What is a Plant-Based Diet?

There has often been some confusion as to whether the plant based diet is just another word for veganism, or if they are a completely different concept with different rules, so let's go into that. There are many similarities between the two, but also some distinct differences. Are veganism and a plant based diet the same thing? The short answer is no. Like I said before, the particular diet that is chosen and the label it is given depends on the individual, and the reason they have chosen to live this lifestyle. Many vegans choose to be so because they disagree with the slaughter and poor treatment of farm animals, and so they do not consume these foods. They also usually choose not to use leather or wear fur or any other animal products. Vegans do not eat any sort of meat, or product containing traces of meat. This includes any broths or ingredients such as gelatin. Vegans also do not eat any food products that contain ANY ingredient from an animal, including milk or honey. They do not eat any cheese, or yogurt, or margarine or butter, etc. Some slightly more hidden ingredients that contain animal products are whey and casein. These are all avoided. Vegans get most of their food from plant sources, but they are not strictly whole food plant based. They may not be as health conscious, and so many may choose to eat packaged and processed foods yet stay away from those made of animals. This technically still falls within the parameter of their diet.

Plant based folks eat a primarily plant derived diet-as close to nature as possible. But this does not mean that they are vegan, or even vegetarian. They may simply choose to eat mostly fruits, vegetables, nuts, and legumes, etc. However, they may still choose to eat meat, and carefully choose meats that are antibiotics free, grass fed, and lived a free range life. Many plant based dieters believe that meat is still an integral part of a healthy diet, and so they just choose the best quality possible.

Whole food, plant based diets usually take the qualities of both diets and even go a step further. Keeping foods whole refers to leaving them in their most natural state. So, vegetables and fruit are eaten as they are-fresh, frozen, or dried without preservatives or added flavor. Nuts are natural, without salt or sugar; grains are not refined or enriched or bleached. Most foods are prepared at home, or in a restaurant where the chefs share the same standards, as to not degrade any of the ingredients or take away any of their nutritional value. Many processed foods use what is known as plant fragments, rather than whole plants. They are reduced or extracted or otherwise processed in some way.

Whatever the specifics of the diet someone chooses, if they tell you that they are vegan or plant based, you should assume that they do not consume any animal products at all, unless they mention it otherwise. This can help you to avoid accidentally serving them something that they will not be willing or able to eat. And feel free to ask someone about their diet, if you are curious. But make sure that they are willing to talk about it, and also that you listen with an open mind- not looking to judge or challenge their decision to adopt that particular diet.

Now, I would like to clarify the way in which I am using the word diet here. I know that many diets are short-term and involve cutting calories and foods in order to lose unwanted weight. This is a bit of a touchy thing because there are many diets out there that can put extreme pressure on the body and will cause weight loss through force or a particular calculation or schedule of eating. This is not what I am referring to in this book. What I will be proposing is that you, the reader, adopt a new addition to your lifestyle that will benefit you, and that you can stick with permanently. This may sound a bit intimidating, to adopt new eating rules for life. However, it is my hope that with my help, you will be able to do this painlessly, and really see benefits from it. You may lose weight; you may have clearer skin and eyes, healthier hair, and even have more abundant energy. And you will help to determine just which benefits you will be rewarded with, by deciding how far you want to go.

Chapter 2: What's plant based diet and why you should try it

Though there are variations within a plant-based diet, the major cornerstone of the diet is that plant foods become the central focal point of your diet. This means that you base your meals around food products sourced from plants like vegetables, nuts, seeds, whole grains, fruits, and legumes. Animal products are either cut out completely or are otherwise reduced. How much you reduce your intake of animal products depends upon what you deem best for yourself. However, if you do choose to make animal products such as fish, poultry, meat, dairy, or eggs a part of your diet, they will take a backseat to the plant foods that make up your meals. If this makes you feel nervous, don't worry! This is not a deprivation diet. There are so many appetizing and tasty plant food options out there that you may not even know about! Many of us are so accustomed to meat, animal products and processed foods taking center-stage at meal times that it is hard to imagine what a meal that puts plant foods first would look like. Embarking on a plant-based diet provides you an exciting opportunity to explore new foods and recipes that are not only satisfying and nourishing but are delicious and taste amazing as well.

The following diets all fall under the umbrella of a plant-based diet:

- *Vegan*: Diet includes vegetables, seeds, nuts, legumes, grains, and fruit and excludes all animal products (i.e. no animal flesh, dairy, or eggs). There are variations within the vegan diet as well such as the *fruitarian* diet made up mainly of fruits and sometimes nuts and seeds and the *raw vegan* diet where food is not cooked.

- *Vegetarian*: Diet includes vegetables, fruit, nuts, legumes, grains, and seeds and excludes meat but may include eggs or dairy. The *Ovo-lacto vegetarian* diet incorporates dairy and eggs while the *Ovo-vegetarian* diet incorporates eggs and excludes dairy and the *lacto vegetarian* diet incorporates dairy but excludes eggs.

- *Semi-vegetarianism:* Diet is mostly vegetarian but also incorporates some meat and animal products. The *macrobiotic* diet is a type of semi-vegetarian diet that emphasizes vegetables, beans, whole grains, naturally processed foods, and may include some seafood, meat, or poultry. The *pescatarian* diet includes plant foods, eggs, dairy, and seafood but no other types of animal flesh. People who subscribe to a semi-vegetarian diet sometimes describe themselves as flexitarians as well. The plant-based, whole food diet is really all about trying to only consume whole, unrefined plants. Followers of a plant-based diet like to get their food as organically as possible. If the food is refined, it must only be minimally refined. Vegetables, fruits, whole grains, tubers, and legumes are going to be the most important parts of meals and animal products either take a on a small proportion of the meal or are excluded altogether. This includes meat, dairy products, and eggs. Highly refined products like bleached flour, oil, and refined sugar are usually avoided as well. Some of these plant-based diets are obviously stricter than others. No one diet is right for everyone, so it is important to understand all the options you have within a plant-based diet so that you can choose which lifestyle is most attractive and feels right to you. Maybe you want to cut out all animal products and go vegan, consuming only plant foods and products or maybe you prefer keeping some animal products in your diet while making plant foods your main focus. Remember, you are in control of what you eat and what goes into your body. A plant-based diet will likely have more restrictions and parameters than you are used to, so it is crucial that you pick a diet that is not only healthy, but attainable, realistic to adhere to, and enjoyable for you. The plant-based diet is designed to increase your quality of life so it would be counter-productive to choose a diet that makes you feel deprived or unhappy! It is important to set realistic expectations for yourself so that you are able to follow your new diet and are not tempted to stray from it. That being said, following a plant-based diet can be incredibly easy and simple if you follow the right steps and stay committed to your new healthy choices which will not be hard to do once you start feeling the beneficial effects of this health-focused lifestyle.

Benefits of Eating a Plant-Based Diet

Plant based diet may lower the risk of cancer and people on vegan diet may have a 15% lower risk of getting cancer or die from it. It can be effective at reducing symptoms of arthritis such as pain, joint swelling and morning stiffness.

Some good news is that a plant-based diet makes your body stronger, so it can resist many types of diseases. Some effects of these diseases can be limited or controlled, while others can be eliminated completely. Now it's your time to change your life!

Weight loss is based on a nutrient-dense diet, and it's all that is needed to achieve your goals. So, if you have been trying to lose weight, now is the time to make that change in your life! Carefully read every section of this cookbook, and you'll get to know what is essential about this plant-based diet. You will find it interesting really. There are several benefits of consuming a plant-based diet. Plants provide three different types of nutrients: macro, micro and phytonutrients. They all work differently and, in conjunction, bring positive effects to human health. Macronutrients ensure a good dose of energy and muscle building, while micronutrients participate in active metabolism. Phytonutrients on the other hand play a role in healing. Experimental evidence suggests that a diet richer in plant-based produce has proven to be more effective and healthier for the human mind and body. Even incurable health disorders are now being cured using nothing but plant-based ingredients. We all know that every plant contains some sort of therapeutic properties. When we add those properties to our daily diet, imagine how much impact it can have on our health outcomes. That is the concept behind the plant-based diet. Not only is it animal-friendly, but it also affects a range of benefits to our health. The oils and fats present in plants are unsaturated and lack bad cholesterol, so they can prevent all heart disorders and cardiac issues. The proteins sourced from plants are less complex and less toxic. Plant sourced carbohydrates are coupled with vitamins, minerals, and fibers. Perhaps a plant-based diet can guarantee a complete, balanced mix of nutrients on a single platter. This cookbook gives you 150 delicious plant-based recipes, bringing this concept of balance one step closer to you so that you can live a healthy, eco-friendly lifestyle.

Since plants offer a balanced mix of all nutrients, it can prevent weight gain. The reduced amount of cholesterol also balances high blood cholesterol levels and consequently controls blood pressure. People suffering from cardiac problems, cancers, high cholesterol, diabetes and obesity are all, therefore, recommended to consume a plant-based, organic diet. According to a meta-analysis of 343 research studies, organic foods consist of 65 percent antioxidants, which can counter the negative effects of cancer and high blood sugar levels in the case of diabetes. While on this diet, every individual can follow a unique diet plan based on their specific health needs.

Chapter 3: What to eat and what to avoid

If you are on a vegan diet you do not have to eat only vegetables and fruits. Lots of usual dishes are already vegan or can be easily turned into vegan. And people that follow the vegan path have a wide variety of options to choose from to substitute animal products. Seitan, tempeh and tofu are versatile protein-rich options that can replace meat, poultry fish and eggs.

Peas, lentils and beans have lots of nutrients and beneficial plant compounds.

Nuts are a perfect choice in terms of fiber, iron, zinc, magnesium, vitamin E and selenium.

Chia, flaxseeds and hemp seeds contain omega-3 fatty acids, and protein.

Plant milks and yogurts help achieve the needed daily calcium intakes.

Chlorella and spirulina have complete protein in them, while other varieties of algae have iodine.

Nutritional yeast has protein in it.

The whole family of whole grains, cereals can help with complex carbohydrates, fiber, iron, B vitamins and various minerals. To get as much protein as possible choose spelt, teff, amaranth and quinoa.

Fruits and vegetables are great choices to increase the nutrient intake.

People that switched to plant-based diet must *avoid*

consuming any animal products and products that have ingredients of animal origin. Meat, poultry and products that contain any meat ingredients.

Fish, seafood and products that contain any seafood ingredients.

Dairy and products that contain any dairy ingredients. Eggs and products that contain any egg ingredients.

Chapter 4: Getting Started

The first thing to be sure of when starting a plant-based diet is that you know what plant foods are going to get you the best bang for your buck. There are a lot of great options out there, but honing in on the most potent (those foods containing the most vitamins, minerals, and nutrients) will really maximize the benefits you are looking to get out of a plant-based diet. So, go for gold and choose the foods that will really make your meals worthwhile. These foods will be like the MVPs (Most Valuable Players) of your new diet. They will help you get the most out of a plant-based diet, make you healthier, and ensure that your food intake is balanced and wholesome. Here are a few Top Ten MVP lists you should keep in mind when planning your plant-based meals:

Vegetables and Legumes

Edamame

These cooked soybeans are not only delicious, but they also have an incredible amount of protein. In just one cup, a serving of edamame will give you 18 g of protein. Look for the certified organic seal, though, because many soybeans in the United States are treated with pesticides or genetically modified. Edamame works great as a stand-alone snack or appetizer and can also be added into meals as a side or in a stir-fry.

Lentils

Easy to incorporate into almost any meal in a variety of forms, lentils provide an excellent source of low-calorie and high-fiber protein. They contain 9 g of protein per half cup serving. They are also incredibly helpful in lowering cholesterol and promoting heart health. You can prepare them as a side dish, use them to make veggie burgers, substitute them for meat and make a delicious taco filling in a slow cooker or make a yummy dip with them.

Black Beans

Black beans are another vegetable like lentils that are wonderfully multi-use. They have great fiber, folate, potassium, and vitamin B6. They contain 7.6 g of protein in every serving and can be used to make anything from veggie burgers to vegan brownies. Imagine that!

Potatoes

Potatoes are a great, low-cost source of protein (4 g per medium potato) and

potassium. They're tasty and heart-healthy!

Spinach

One of the best green vegetables for protein (3 g per serving), cooked spinach is an excellent addition to your plant-based diet.

Broccoli

When cooked, you get 2 g per serving of this vegetable and also an excellent dose of fiber.

Brussels Sprouts

Another great green vegetable for protein, brussels sprouts gives you 2 g of protein per serving alongside a great deal of potassium and vitamin K. Be sure to get the fresh version, though, as they taste a whole lot better than the frozen kind!

Lima Beans

Containing 7.3 g of protein per serving when cooked, lima beans make an amazing side dish or addition to a healthy salad. They also contain leucine, an amino acid that aids in muscle synthesis

Peanuts and Peanut Butter

Widely recognized as a superfood by meat-eaters and plant-based eaters alike, peanuts and peanut butter contain 7 g of protein per serving and can be used in so many different ways. And who doesn't love a good childhood staple PB&J sandwich? Nearly all kinds of peanut butter are vegan but keep a lookout for any that might contain honey if you are keeping strictly vegan and cutting out all animal products.

Chickpeas

Chickpeas are another versatile legume that can be prepared in a multitude of ways. Perhaps the most popular preparation is in the form of delicious hummus. With 6 g of protein per serving, it'll be hard not to spread it on everything you eat!

Nuts and Seeds

Chia Seeds

Chia seeds are amazing sources of vitamin C, protein, fiber, and calcium. They have to be soaked in liquid and allowed to expand. Once properly prepared, you can sprinkle them on top of almost anything!

Pumpkin Seeds

Pumpkin seeds work great for a tasty and easy snack and can also be added to salads, yogurt, and soups. They pack a lot of great nutrients like Vitamins C, E, and K, omega-3 fatty acids, and iron in a small package.

Almonds

Commonly considered nuts, almonds are more accurately categorized as a fruit of the almond tree. They are wonderful sources of fiber, protein, magnesium, phosphorus, calcium, potassium, iron, and B vitamins. Like soybeans, they are often used in dairy substitutes and they have been shown to lower cholesterol, strengthen bones, and promote a healthy cardiovascular system. Plus, they are great for your skin and hair!

Flaxseeds

Flaxseeds are great additives to plant-based meals. They can be ground up and added to smoothies, oatmeal, cereal, or baked into muffins, bread, and cookies. They are high in protein, magnesium, zinc, and B vitamins. They also aid in digestion and help with weight loss by suppressing appetite.

Walnuts

These nuts are some of the best natural sources of omega-3 fatty acids. They also contain plenty of vitamin E, protein, calcium, zinc, and potassium. These, like many of the other nuts and seeds on this list, can be enjoyed alone as a snack or added to other dishes.

Sesame Seeds

Sesame seeds are a great natural way to lower cholesterol and high blood pressure and can also help with afflictions like migraines, arthritis, and asthma. They are great in bread and crackers and can be used in stir-fry meals and salads.

Sunflower Seeds

These seeds are great for vitamin E and contain healthy fats, B vitamins, and iron. They can be eaten dry and are also used to make butter, a great alternative to dairy.

Cashews

Though cashews, like almonds, are not technically nuts and are rather the fruit of the cashew tree, they are most commonly treated as nuts. With their low sodium content and great flavor, they are a popular source of protein and vitamins.

Brazil Nuts

These delicious nuts from the Bertholletia excelsa tree mature inside a large coconut-like shell. They are wonderful for protein, fiber, iron, and many B-complex vitamins.

Pine Nuts

Pine nuts contain great antioxidants as well as lots of iron, magnesium, and potassium. They are low in calories and go wonderfully with many dishes. You can use them in baked foods or add them in sauces like an Italian pesto.

Whole Grains

Quinoa

Quinoa certainly has made a splash onto the health food scene with countless people boasting about its beneficial qualities. Although it is actually a seed, we treat it mainly as a grain in the way in which it is prepared. This South American gem has an incredible amount of protein and omega-3 fatty acids and is an important staple of anyone looking to get more of these nutrients within a plant-based diet. It can be used in a multitude of dishes and is as versatile as it is healthy!

Wheat

A classic staple, whole wheat is incredibly beneficial to your health. Each serving of whole grain has about 2 to 3 g of fiber which is a great way to make sure your body is functioning healthily and properly. Be sure to steer clear of multi-grain, however, and go for the stuff marked 100% whole grain to make sure you are getting exactly what you need!

Oats

These whole grains are packed full of heart-healthy antioxidants. Oats are great and can be enjoyed as a fulfilling breakfast in the form of oatmeal and they can also be ground up and used as a healthier flour substitute when baking. Unsweetened oats are the best to buy and if you are craving a little something sugary, throw in a few berries or a dollop of honey if you wish.

Brown Rice

Brown rice is incredibly high in antioxidants and good vitamins. It's relative, white rice is far less beneficial as much of these healthy nutrients get destroyed during the process of milling. You can also opt for red and black rice or wild rice. The meal options for this healthy grain are limitless!

Rye

Rye is an amazing whole grain that contains four times the fiber of regular whole wheat and gives you almost 50% of day-to-day recommended iron intake. When shopping for rye, however, be sure to look for the whole rye marking as a lot of what is on the market is made with refined flour, thus cutting the benefits in half.

Barley

This whole grain is a miracle food for lowering high cholesterol. It can be quick-cooked like oats and serves as a delicious side dish. You can add whatever kind of toppings you desire to give it your own personal flair! Be sure again to seek out the whole-grain barley as other types may have the bran or germ removed.

Buckwheat

Buckwheat is a great gluten-free grain option for those with celiac disease or a gluten intolerance. It's a great source of magnesium and manganese. Buckwheat is used to make delicious gluten free pancakes and easily becomes a morning staple!

Bulgur

This grain is a truly excellent source of iron and magnesium. It also contains a wonderful amount of protein and fiber with one cup containing about 75% of daily recommended fiber and 25% or daily recommended protein. It goes great in salads and soups and is easy to cook. Talk about amazing!

Couscous

This grain is another great source of fiber. A lot of the couscous you see in the store will be made from refined flour, though, so it is important that you seek out the whole wheat kind so that you can get all the healthy, yummy benefits.

Corn

Whole corn is a fantastic source of phosphorus, magnesium, and B vitamins. It also promotes healthy digestion and contains heart-healthy antioxidants. It is important to seek out organic corn in order to bypass all the genetically modified product that is out on the market.

Fruits

Avocado

Widely acknowledged as an incredibly beneficial and healthy super-fruit, avocados truly are miracle fruits. They are the best way possible to get the kind of substantial serving of healthy monounsaturated fatty acids that many people subscribing to a plant-based diet seek to supplement. They also contain about 20 different vitamins and minerals and are packed with important nutrients. On top of that, they taste amazing and go well with almost any dish, breakfast, lunch, or dinner!

Grapefruit

Grapefruits are packed full of Vitamin C, containing much more than oranges. Half a grapefruit provides you with almost 50% of your recommended daily vitamin C. It also gives you incredible levels of Vitamin A, fiber, and potassium. It can help with afflictions like arthritis and is a great remedy for oily skin.

Pineapple

This fruit can be prepared and enjoyed in a variety of ways making it not only a tasty and fun treat but also a great healthy choice! It is full of anti-inflammatory nutrients that can help reduce the risk of stroke or heart attack. Some studies show that it also increases fertility.

Blueberries

These little berries not only taste delicious and go with so many different dishes, they are also full of vitamin C and healthful antioxidants. Studies also show that it promotes eye health and can slow macular degeneration which causes older adults to go blind.

Pomegranate

Whether in juice form or seed, consuming pomegranate is a great way to get potassium. It has fantastic antioxidants (three times more than green tea or red wine) that work to promote cardiovascular and heart health as well as lower cholesterol levels

Apple

The old saying "an apple a day keeps the doctor away" is not just an old wives' tale! It is low-calorie and incredibly healthy. Apples contain antioxidants that protect brain cell health and are heart-healthy. They can also lower high cholesterol and aid in weight loss and healthy teeth.

Kiwi

This tart, delicious fruit is not only unique but also full of great vitamins like C and E. These are powerful antioxidants that some studies show help with eye health and can even lower chances of cancer. They are low-calorie and very high in fiber. This makes them great for aiding in weight loss and they make a wonderful, quick, easy, and guilt-free snack.

Mango

Mangoes have excellent levels of the nutrient beta-carotene. The body converts this into Vitamin A which in turn strengthens bone health and the immune system. They also have a huge amount of Vitamin C-50% of the daily recommended value to be exact.

Lemons

Everyone knows that lemons and other citrus fruit are high in Vitamin C, however, they are also an excellent source of antioxidants, fiber, and folate. Lemons can help lower cholesterol, the risk of some kinds of cancer, and blood pressure. All at just 17 calories a serving!

Cranberries

Cranberries are another fruit that have more than one health benefit. They have great vitamin C and fiber levels and have more antioxidants than many other fruits and vegetables. At only 45 calories a serving, it is a great way to boost your immune system, keep your urinary tract healthy, and absorb other important nutrients like Vitamins E, K, and manganese.

Armed with these plant food MVPs, you can begin to make your transition into a healthy, delicious plant-based diet. Incorporating these foods into your diet will help you build balanced meals that will give you the energy and sustenance you need to go about your day. All of these top ten MVPs are incredibly healthy so you can indulge in them guilt-free because you know that they are giving you so many valuable vitamins, minerals, antioxidants, and other nutrients. Many of these foods are low in calories as well and have amazing health benefits like lowering high cholesterol and promoting a healthy heart and cardiovascular system. If you keep these MVPs in mind, you really cannot go wrong. And as a bonus, there is so much room for creative meal opportunities that are bursting not only with flavor but also with amazing health benefits.

So, how do you transition into a plant-based diet? The easy answer is gradually. Remember, slow and steady always wins the race, every time. Though it is positive, there is no diminishing the fact that this will be a big change for you, especially if you have become used to consuming a lot of animal products and processed foods. Things may feel different and unfamiliar at first, so it is natural to be hesitant. But in reality, transitioning into a plant-based diet is not a scary thing. You can start small! Begin by slowly adding more vegetables, beans, fruits, whole grains, seeds, and nuts to your diet. Here are a few suggestions:

• Make a grocery list that incorporates at least two items from each of our four MVP lists mentioned above. Lists are a great way to get motivated and stay on task; color coordination never goes astray either. Make the list aesthetically appealing or even turn it into a chart and start tracking what items you've tried, liked and will repurchase and what items you'll try next grocery shop.

• Slowly start clearing out your pantry, cupboards and fridge of processed, unhealthy foods so you aren't tempted to snack on them when at home and replace them with healthy substitutes (below we will discuss some fantastic alternatives). You may keep one or two indulgences to begin with as you slowly wean yourself off sweets and retrain your mind.

• Try to incorporate two or three of our MVPs into your dinner each night even if it's a small proportion to begin with.

You might start with these foods as a side dish and slowly build up to surrounding your meals around them. You could begin the transition with MVP Mondays and make a delicious meal especially on these nights packed with valuable nutrients – a good way to start the week!

• Try something different for dessert! If you must snack after dinner try some fruits as they are sure to satisfy your sugar cravings, have some blueberries, pomegranates or strawberries with some delicious coconut yoghurt.

• Make your lunch for work, either the night before (or morning of if you have time) and restrict yourself to only buying lunch once a week as a treat. This will enable you to understand exactly what's going into your body and eliminate the need to play that guessing game: *what exactly was in the mysterious lasagna from the café?!*

• Start taking little containers to work full of nuts or cut up fruit and leaving them on your desk or in your bag to pick at whenever you feel a little hungry. This is a great way to train your mind to stop thinking 'snack' means junk food, it does not have to, and I ensure you your energy levels will rise.

This will help you get familiar with plant-based food products and start to make them a staple in your day to day consumptions. Slowly but surely the sugar cravings will diminish as you cleanse your body with whole foods. Tailor your plant-based choices to your specific likes, but don't be afraid to be a little adventurous and try something new! There are so many wonderful and exciting plant-based foods to try. If you browse your local health food market, it is inevitable that you will come across something you have not yet consumed. Make a little pact with yourself that you will try a new plant-based food every week or every two weeks. See what works for you. You never know, you may just discover your new favorite food!

Chapter 5: Breakfast

1. **Apple Pancakes**

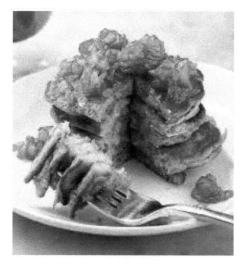

Preparation Time: 15 Minutes
Cooking time: 4 minutes
Servings: 4

Ingredients:

1 cup whole-wheat flour

¾ tsp. ground cinnamon, divided

¼ tsp. baking soda

1 tsp. baking powder

Pinch salt

1 egg

¾ cup ricotta cheese

1 cup buttermilk

1 tsp. vanilla extract

1 tbsp. sugar and 1 tsp. sugar, divided

1 apple, sliced into rings

4 tsp. butter

4 tsp. walnut oil

Direction:

In a bowl, mix the flour, ½ teaspoon cinnamon, baking soda, baking powder and salt.

In another bowl, beat the eggs and stir in the cheese, milk, vanilla and 1 tablespoon sugar.

Gradually add the second bowl to the first one. Mix well.

Combine the remaining cinnamon and 1 teaspoon sugar in a separate dish.

Coat each apple ring with this mixture.

Pour the butter and oil in a pan over medium heat.

Add the apples and pour the batter around the apple. Cook for 2 minutes.

Flip and cook for another 2 minutes.

<u>Nutrition</u>: Calories 342, Total Fat 16 g, Saturated Fat 7 g, Cholesterol 83 mg, Sodium 448 mg, Total Carbohydrate 38 g, Dietary Fiber 4g, Protein 13 g, Total Sugars 12 g, Potassium 252 mg

2. Cream Cheese Waffles

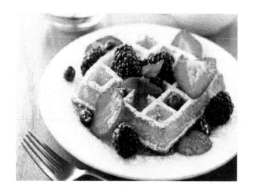

Preparation Time: 5 Minutes

Cooking time: 0 minute

Serving: 1

Ingredients:

1 whole-grain waffle

1 tbsp. cream cheese

1 tbsp. granola

1 plum, sliced

Direction:

Toast the waffle. Place it on a plate. Spread the top with cream cheese.

Arrange granola and plum and serve.

Nutrition: Calories 188, Total Fat 10 g, Saturated Fat 4 g, Cholesterol 15 mg, Sodium 219 mg, Total Carbohydrate 25 g, Dietary Fiber 5 g, Protein 4 g, Total Sugars 10 g, Potassium 225 mg.

3. Herb & Cheese Omelet

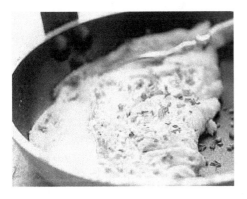

Preparation Time: 5 Minutes

Cooking time: 5 minutes

Servings: 2

Ingredients:

4 eggs

Salt and pepper to taste

2 tbsp. low-fat milk

1 tsp. chives, chopped

1 tbsp. parsley, chopped

½ cup goat cheese, crumbled

1 tsp. olive oil

Direction: Beat the eggs in a bowl.

Stir in the salt, pepper and milk.

In a bowl, combine the chives, parsley and goat cheese.

Pour the oil into a pan over medium heat.

Cook the eggs for 3 minutes.

Add the cheese mixture on top.

Fold and serve.

Nutrition: Calories 227, Total Fat 17 g, Saturated Fat 7 g, Cholesterol 397 mg, Sodium 386 mg, Total Carbohydrate 3 g, Dietary Fiber 1 g, Protein 17 g, Total Sugars 1 g, Potassium 183 mg

4. Pineapple Bagel with Cream Cheese

Preparation Time: 10 Minutes

Cooking time: 3 minutes

Servings: 8

Ingredients:

8 pineapple slices

4 tsp. brown sugar

4 whole-wheat bagels, sliced in half and toasted

6 oz. cream cheese

3 tbsp. almonds, toasted and sliced

Direction:

Preheat your broiler.

Line your baking pan with parchment paper.

Place the pineapple slices on the baking pan

Sprinkle each with the sugar.

Broil the pineapples for 3 minutes.

Spread the cream cheese on top of the bagels.

Sprinkle almonds on top. Top each bagel with the pineapple slices.

Nutrition: Calories 157, Total Fat 6 g, Saturated Fat 3 g, Cholesterol 16 mg,

Sodium 167 mg, Total Carbohydrate 23 g, Dietary Fiber 4g, Protein 6 g, Total Sugars 10 g, Potassium 110 mg

5. Scrambled Eggs with Spinach

Preparation Time: 5 Minutes

Cooking time: 4 minutes

Servings: 2

Ingredients:

2 tsp. olive oil

3 cups baby spinach

4 eggs, beaten

Salt and pepper to taste

2 slices whole-wheat bread, toasted

1 cup raspberries, sliced

Direction:

Pour the olive oil into a pan over medium heat.

Cook the spinach for 2 minutes.

Transfer to a plate.

Add the eggs to the pan.

Cook while stirring frequently for 2 minutes.

Add the spinach and season with salt and pepper.

Serve scrambled egg on top of the bread, and with raspberries.

Nutrition: Calories 296, Total Fat 16 g, Saturated Fat 4 g, Cholesterol 372 mg, Sodium 394 mg, Total Carbohydrate 21 g, Dietary Fiber 7 g, Protein 18 g, Total Sugars 5 g, Potassium 293 mg

6. Oatmeal Pancake

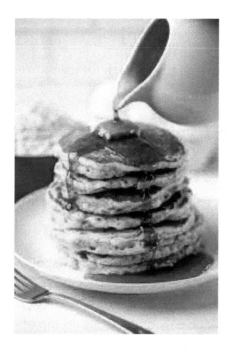

Preparation Time: 10 Minutes

Cooking time: 30 minutes

Servings: 8

Ingredients:

½ cup blueberries

3 bananas, sliced

2 tsp. lemon juice

¼ cup maple syrup

¼ tsp. ground cinnamon

1 cup flour

2 tsp. baking powder

½ tsp. baking soda

½ cup rolled oats

Salt to taste

1 egg, beaten

1 cup buttermilk

1 tsp. vanilla

1 tbsp. olive oil

Direction:

Toss the blueberries and bananas in lemon juice, maple syrup and cinnamon. Set aside.

In a bowl, mix the flour, baking powder, baking soda, oats and salt.

In another bowl, combine the egg, milk and vanilla.

Slowly add the second bowl mixture into the first one. Mix well.

Pour the oil into a pan over medium heat.

Pour 4 tablespoons of the batter and cook for 2 minutes per side.

Repeat with the remaining batter.

Serve the pancakes with the fruits.

Nutrition: Calories 159, Total Fat 3 g, Saturated Fat 0 g, Cholesterol 1 mg, Sodium 246 mg, Total Carbohydrate 31 g, Dietary Fiber 2 g, Protein 5 g, Total Sugars
 8 g, Potassium 260 mg

7. **Waffles with Pumpkin & Cream Cheese**

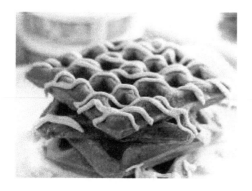

Preparation Time: 5 Minutes

Cooking time: 1 minute

Serving: 1

Ingredients:

1 whole-wheat waffle

½ oz. cream cheese

1 tbsp. canned pumpkin puree

1 tsp. walnuts, toasted and chopped

Direction:

Toast the waffle.

Mix the cream cheese and pumpkin.

Spread the mixture on top of the waffle.

Sprinkle the walnuts on top.

Nutrition: Calories 132 Total Fat 7 g, Saturated Fat 2 g, Cholesterol 10 mg, Sodium 203 mg, Total Carbohydrate 14 g Dietary Fiber 4g, Protein 4 g, Total Sugars 2 g, Potassium 310 mg

8. Avocado & Egg Salad on Toasted Bread

Preparation Time: 5 Minutes

Cooking time: 0 minute

Servings: 2

Ingredients:

½ avocado

1 tsp. lemon juice

2 hard-boiled egg, chopped

2 tbsp. celery, chopped

Salt to taste

1 tsp. hot sauce

2 slices whole-wheat bread, toasted

Direction:

Mash the avocado in a bowl.

Stir in the lemon juice, egg, celery, salt and hot sauce.

Spread the mixture on top of the toasted bread.

Nutrition:

Calories 230, Total Fat 14 g, Saturated Fat 3 g, Cholesterol 186 mg, Sodium 405 mg, Total Carbohydrate 17 g

Dietary Fiber 5g, Protein 11g, Total Sugars 2g, Potassium 400mg

9. Cottage Cheese, Honey & Raspberries

Preparation Time: 10 Minutes

Cooking time: 0 minute

Servings: 4

Ingredients:

2 cups fresh raspberries

1 tsp. lemon zest

2 tbsp. honey

2 cups cottage cheese

2 tbsp. sunflower seeds, roasted

Direction:

Add 1 cup raspberry in your food processor.

Pulse until pureed.

Transfer to a bowl and stir in the lemon zest and honey.

Divide the cottage cheese among 4 bowls.

Top each one with the raspberry mixture.

Nutrition:

Calories 169, Total Fat 4 g, Saturated Fat 1 g, Cholesterol 5 mg

Sodium 476 mg, Total Carbohydrate 20 g, Dietary Fiber 4g, Protein 16 g, Total Sugars 15 g, Potassium 230 mg

Chapter 6: Soups, Salads and Sides

10. Butternut Squash Soup

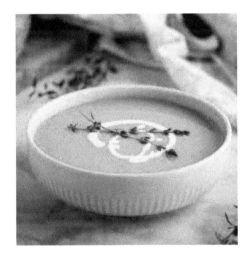

Preparation Time: 15 Minutes

Cooking time: 25 minutes

Servings: 6

Ingredients:

2 tbsp. olive oil

1 cup onion, chopped

1 cup cilantro

1 ginger, sliced thinly

2 cups pears, chopped

½ tsp. ground coriander

Salt to taste

2 ½ lb. butternut squash, cubed

1 tsp. lime zest

26 oz. coconut milk

1 tbsp. lime juice

½ cup plain yogurt

Direction:

Pour the oil into a pan over medium heat.

Add the onion, cilantro, ginger, pears, coriander and salt.

Stir and cook for 5 minutes.

Transfer to a pressure cooker.

Stir in the squash and lime zest.

Pour in the coconut milk.

Cook on high for 20 minutes.

Release pressure naturally.

Stir in the lime juice.

Transfer to a blender.

Pulse until smooth.

Reheat and stir in yogurt
before serving.

Nutrition: Calories 274, Total
Fat 14 g, Saturated Fat 8 g,
Cholesterol 3 mg, Sodium 438
mg, Total Carbohydrate 36 g,
Dietary Fiber 6 g, Protein 5 g,
Total Sugars 11 g, Potassium
715 mg

11. Lemon & Strawberry Soup

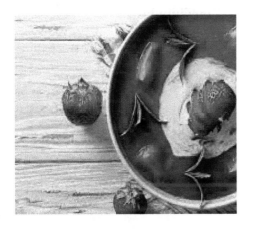

Preparation Time: 4 hours and 10 Minutes

Cooking time: 0 minute

Servings: 4

Ingredients:

1 cup buttermilk

3 cups strawberries, sliced

1 tsp. lemon thyme

2 tsp. lemon zest

2 tbsp. honey

Direction:

Blend the buttermilk and strawberries in your food processor.

Transfer this mixture to a bowl.

Add the thyme and lemon zest.

Chill in the refrigerator for 4 hours.

Strain the soup and stir in the honey.

Serve in bowls.

Nutrition:

Calories 92, Total Fat 1 g, Saturated Fat 0 g, Cholesterol 2 mg, Sodium 66 mg

Total Carbohydrate 20 g, Dietary Fiber 2 g, Protein 3 g, Total Sugars 17 g, Potassium 266 mg

12. Tomato Soup with Kale & White Beans

Preparation Time: 5 Minutes

Cooking time: 7 minutes

Servings: 4

Ingredients:

28 oz. tomato soup

1 tbsp. olive oil

3 cups kale, chopped

14 oz. cannellini beans, rinsed and drained

1 tsp. garlic, crushed and minced

¼ cup Parmesan cheese, grated

Direction:

Pour the soup into a pan over medium heat.

Add the oil and cook the kale for 2 minutes.

Stir in the beans and garlic.

Simmer for 5 minutes.

Sprinkle with Parmesan cheese before serving.

Nutrition: Calories 200, Total Fat 6 g, Saturated Fat 1 g, Cholesterol 4 mg, Sodium 355 mg, Total Carbohydrate 29 g, Dietary Fiber 6 g, Protein 9 g, Total Sugars 1 g, Potassium 257 mg

13. Bursting Black Bean Soup

Servings: 6

Preparation time: 8 hours and 10 minutes

Ingredients:

1 pound of black beans, uncooked

1/4 cup of lentils, uncooked

1 medium-sized carrot, peeled and chopped

2 medium-sized green bell peppers, cored and chopped

1 stalk of celery, chopped

28 ounce of diced tomatoes

2 jalapeno pepper, seeded and minced

1 large red onion, peeled and chopped

3 teaspoons of minced garlic

1 tablespoon of salt

1/2 teaspoon ground black pepper

2 tablespoons of red chili powder

2 teaspoons of ground cumin

1/2 teaspoon of dried oregano

3 tablespoons of apple cider vinegar

1/2 cup of brown rice, uncooked

3 quarts of water, divided

Direction:

Place a large pot over medium-high heat, add the beans, pour in 1 1/2 quarts of water and boil it.

Let it boil for 10 minutes, then remove the pot from the heat, let it stand for 1 hour and then cover the pot.

Drain the beans and add it to a 6-quarts slow cooker.

Pour in the remaining 1 1/2 quarts of water and cover it with the lid.

Plug in the slow cooker and let it cook for 3 hours at the high setting or until it gets soft.

When the beans are done, add the remaining ingredients except for the rice and continue cooking for 3 hours on the low heat setting.

When it is 30 minutes left to finish, add the rice to the slow cooker and let it cook.   When done, using an immersion blender process half of the soup and then serve.

Nutrition: Calories:116 Cal, Carbohydrates:19g, Protein:5.6g, Fats:1.5g, Fiber:4g

14. Yummy Lentil Rice Soup

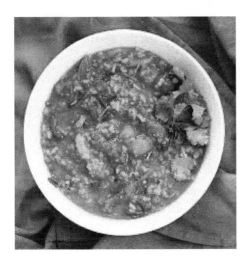

Servings: 6

Preparation time: 4 hours and 15 minutes

Ingredients:

2 cups of brown rice, uncooked

2 cups of lentils, uncooked

1/2 cup of chopped celery

1 cup of chopped carrots

1 cup of sliced mushrooms

1/2 of a medium-sized white onion, peeled and chopped

1 teaspoon of minced garlic

1 tablespoon of salt

1/2 teaspoon of ground black pepper

1 cup of vegetable broth

8 cups of water

Direction:

Using a 6-quarts slow cooker, place all the ingredients except for mushrooms and stir until it mixes properly.

Cover with lid, plug in the slow cooker and let it cook for 3 to 4 hours at the high setting or until it is cooked thoroughly.

Pour in the mushrooms, stir and continue cooking for 1 hour at the low heat setting or until it is done.

Serve right away.

Nutrition: Calories:226 Cal, Carbohydrates:41g,Protein:13g, Fats:2g, Fiber:12g.

15. Tangy Corn Chowder

Servings: 6

Preparation time: 5 hours and 15 minutes

Ingredients:

24 ounce of cooked kernel corn

3 medium-sized potatoes, peeled and diced

2 red chile peppers, minced

1 large white onion, peeled and diced

1 teaspoon of minced garlic

2 teaspoons of salt

1/2 teaspoon of ground black pepper

1 tablespoon of red chili powder

1 tablespoon of dried parsley

1/4 cup of vegan margarine

14 fluid ounce of soy milk

1 lime, juiced

24 fluid ounce of vegetable broth

Direction:

Using a 6-quarts slow cooker place all the ingredients except for the soy milk, margarine, and lime juice.

Stir properly and cover it with the lid.

Then plug in the slow cooker and let it cook for 3 to 4 hours at the high setting or until it is cooked thoroughly.

When done, process the mixture with an immersion blender or until it gets smooth.

Pour in the milk, margarine and stir properly.

Continue cooking the soup for 1 hour at the low heat setting.

Drizzle it with the lime juice and serve.

Nutrition:

Calories:237 Cal,
Carbohydrates:18g,
Protein:7.4g, Fats:15g,
Fiber:2.2g.

16. Healthy Cabbage Soup

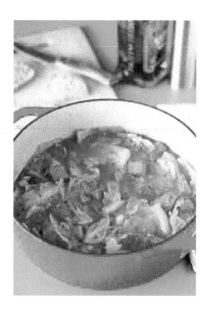

Servings: 6

Preparation time: 4 hours and 15 minutes

Ingredients:

5 cups of shredded cabbage

3 medium-sized carrots, peeled and chopped

3 1/2 cups of diced tomatoes

1 medium-sized white onion, chopped

2 teaspoons of minced garlic

1 teaspoon of salt

1 teaspoon of dried oregano

1 tablespoon of dried parsley

1 1/2 cups of tomato sauce

5 cups of vegetable broth

Direction:

Using a 6-quarts slow cooker, place all the ingredients and stir properly.

Cover it with the lid, plug in the slow cooker and let it cook for 4 hours at the high heat setting or until the vegetables are tender.

Serve right away.

Nutrition:

Calories:150 Cal, Carbohydrates:4g, Protein:20g, Fats:5g, Fiber:2g

17. Eggplant Salad

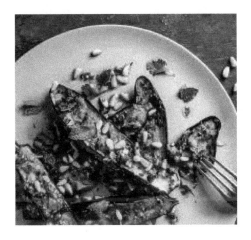

Servings: 6

Preparation Time: 15 minutes

Cooking time: 25 minutes

Ingredient:

2 eggplants

1 teaspoon salt

1 white onion, diced

1 teaspoon Pink salt

1 oz fresh cilantro

3 tablespoon lemon juice

4 tablespoon olive oil

1 garlic clove, peeled

Direction:

Cut eggplants into halves.

Preheat oven to 365F.

Put eggplants in the oven and cook for 25 minutes or until they are tender.

Meanwhile, blend diced onion and transfer in the cheesecloth. Pour olive oil and lemon juice in the bowl.

Squeeze blended onion in the oil mixture. Add salt.

Chop cilantro and grind garlic. Add ingredients in the oily mixture too. Stir it.

Remove the eggplants from the oven and chill them little.

Remove the flesh from the eggplants and transfer in the salad bowl. Add oil mixture and stir gently.

Nutrition: calories 137, fat 9.8, fiber 7, carbs 13, protein 2.2

18. Tricolore Salad

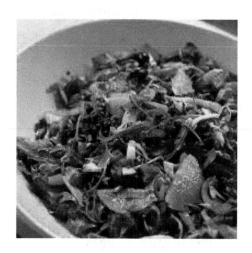

Preparation Time: 10 minutes

Servings:5

Ingredients:

1 avocado, peeled

½ cup kalamata olives

2 tablespoon olive oil

1 teaspoon minced garlic

¼ teaspoon salt

2 tomatoes, chopped

1 teaspoon apple cider vinegar

6 oz Provolone cheese, chopped

Direction:
 Mix up together salt, apple cider vinegar, minced garlic, and olive oil.

Cut kalamata olives into halves.

Slice avocado and place in salad bowl.

Add olive halves, chopped tomato, and cheese.

Stir gently and sprinkle with olive oil mixture.

Nutrition: calories 275, fat 24, fiber 3.7, carbs 7.1, protein 10

19. "Potato" Salad

Servings: 4

Preparation Time: 10 minutes

Cooking time: 15 minutes

Ingredients:

8 oz turnip, peeled

1 carrot, peeled

1 bay leaf

¼ teaspoon peppercorns

1 teaspoon salt

½ teaspoon cayenne pepper

1 tablespoon fresh parsley, chopped

3 eggs, boiled

3 tablespoon sour cream

1 tablespoon mustard

2 cups water, for vegetables

Direction:

Put turnip and carrot in the saucepan.

Add water, peppercorns, bay leaf, and salt.

Close the lid and boil vegetables for 15 minutes over high heat. The cooked vegetables should be tender.

Meanwhile, peel eggs and chop them.

Put the chopped eggs in the bowl.

Sprinkle them with cayenne pepper and chopped parsley.

In the separate bowl stir together mustard and sour cream.

When the vegetables are cooked, strain them and transfer in the salad bowl. Add mustard sauce and stir.

Nutrition: calories 104, fat 6.1, fiber 2, carbs 7.2, protein 5.9

20. Florentine

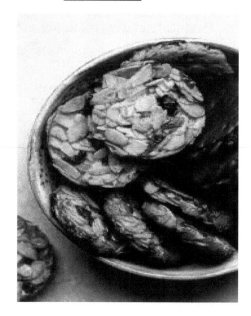

Servings: 4

Preparation Time: 10 minutes

Cooking time: 15

Ingredients:

1 teaspoon butter

4 eggs

8 oz Edam cheese, shredded

1 teaspoon ground paprika

¼ teaspoon cayenne pepper

2 tablespoon cream cheese

Direction:

Preheat oven to 360F.

Preheat the springform pan in the oven.

Then grease it with butter.

Beat the eggs in the greased pan and sprinkle with cayenne pepper.

Top eggs with shredded cheese and spread with cream cheese.

Sprinkle the meal with ground paprika.

Put it in the oven and cook for 15 minutes or until cheese is light brown at 355F.

Nutrition: calories 293, fat 22.9, fiber 0.2, carbs 1.6, protein 20.2

21. Chunky Potato Soup

Servings: 6

Preparation time: 6 hours and 10 minutes

Ingredients:

1 medium-sized carrot, grated

6 medium-sized potatoes, peeled and diced

2 stalks of celery, diced

1 medium-sized white onion, peeled and diced

2 teaspoons of minced garlic

1 1/2 teaspoons of salt

1 teaspoon of ground black pepper

1 1/2 teaspoons of dried sage

1 teaspoon of dried thyme

2 tablespoons of olive oil

2 bay leaves

8 1/2 cups of vegetable water

Direction:

Using a 6-quarts slow cooker, place all the ingredients and stir properly.

Cover it with the lid, plug in the slow cooker and let it cook for 6 hours at the high heat setting or until the potatoes are tender.

Serve right away.

Nutrition: Calories:200 Cal, Carbohydrates:26g, Protein:6g, Fats:8g, Fiber:2g.

22. Yogurt Soup with Rice

Servings: 6

Preparation Time: 15 minutes

Cooking time: 48 minutes

Ingredients:

½ cup brown rice, rinsed and drained

1 egg

4 cups yogurt

3 tbsp. rice flour

3 cups water

½ cup mint, chopped

½ cup cilantro, chopped

½ cup dill, chopped

½ cup parsley, chopped

2 cups arugula

Salt to taste

Direction:

Combine the rice, egg, yogurt and flour in a pot.

Put it over medium heat and cook for 1 minute, stirring frequently.

Pour in the water and increase heat to boil.

Reduce heat and simmer for 45 minutes.

Add the arugula, herbs and salt.

Cook for 2 minutes.

Add more water to adjust consistency.

Nutrition: Calories 186, Total Fat 7 g, Saturated Fat 4 g, Cholesterol 52 mg, Sodium 486 mg, Total Carbohydrate 24 g, Dietary Fiber 2g, Protein 9g, Total Sugars 8g, Potassium 365 mg

23. Zucchini Soup

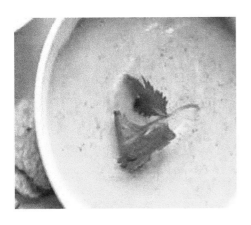

Preparation Time: 5 Minutes

Cooking time: 15 minutes

Servings: 4

Ingredients:

3 cups chicken broth

1 tbsp. tarragon, chopped

3 zucchinis, sliced

3 oz. cheddar cheese

Salt and pepper to taste

Direction:

Pour the broth into a pot.

Stir in the tarragon and zucchini.

Bring to a boil and then simmer for 10 minutes.

Transfer to a blender and blend until smooth.

Put it back to the stove and stir in cheese.

Season with salt and pepper.

Nutrition: Calories 110, Total Fat 5 g, Saturated Fat 3 g, Cholesterol 15 mg, Sodium 757 mg, Total Carbohydrate 7 g, Dietary Fiber 2 g, Protein 10 g, Total Sugars 4g, Potassium 606 mg

24. Cauliflower & Apple Salad

Servings: 4

Preparation Time: 25 Minutes

Ingredients:

3 Cups Cauliflower, Chopped into Florets

2 Cups Baby Kale

1 Sweet Apple, Cored & Chopped

¼ Cup Basil, Fresh & Chopped

¼ Cup Mint, Fresh & Chopped

¼ Cup Parsley, Fresh & Chopped

1/3 Cup Scallions, Sliced Thin

2 Tablespoons Yellow Raisins

1 Tablespoon Sun Dried Tomatoes, Chopped

½ Cup Miso Dressing, Optional

¼ Cup Roasted Pumpkin Seeds, Optional

Direction:

Combine everything together, tossing before serving.

Nutrition: Calories: 198, Protein: 7 g, Fat: 8 g, Carbs: 32 g

Interesting Facts: This vegetable is an extremely high source of vitamin A, vitamin B1, B2 and B3.

25. Corn & Black Bean Salad

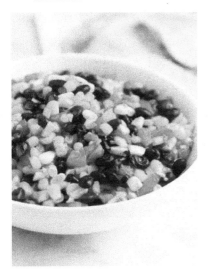

Salad: 6

Preparation Time: 10 Minutes

Ingredients:

¼ Cup Cilantro, Fresh & Chopped

1 Can Corn, Drained (10 Ounces)

1/8 Cup Red Onion, Chopped

1 Can Black Beans, Drained (15 Ounces)

1 Tomato, Chopped

3 Tablespoons Lemon Juice, Fresh

2 Tablespoons Olive Oil

Sea Salt & Black Pepper to Taste

Direction:

Mix everything together, and then refrigerate until cool. Serve cold.

Nutrition: Calories: 159, Protein: 6.4 gFat: 5.6 g, Carbs: 23.7 g

Interesting Facts: Whole corn is a fantastic source of phosphorus, magnesium, and B vitamins. It also promotes healthy digestion and contains heart-healthy antioxidants. It is important to seek out organic corn in order to bypass all of the genetically modified product that is out on the market.

26. Spinach & Orange Salad

Servings: 6

Preparation Time: 15 Minutes

Ingredients:

¼ -1/3 Cup Vegan Dressing

3 Oranges, Medium, Peeled, Seeded & Sectioned

¾ lb. Spinach, Fresh & Torn

1 Red Onion, Medium, Sliced & Separated into Rings

Direction:

Toss everything together and serve with dressing.

Nutrition: Calories: 99, Protein: 2.5 g, Fat: 5 g, Carbs: 13.1 g

Interesting Facts: Spinach is one of the most superb green veggies out there. Each serving is packed with 3 grams of protein and is a highly encouraged component of the plant-based diet.

27. Red Pepper & Broccoli Salad

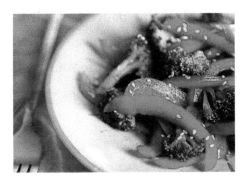

½ Teaspoon Black Pepper

½ Teaspoon Sea Salt, Fine

2 Tablespoons Olive Oil

1 Tablespoon Parsley, Chopped

Servings: 2

Preparation Time: 15 Minutes

Ingredients:

Ounces Lettuce Salad Mix

1 Head Broccoli, Chopped into Florets

1 Red Pepper, Seeded & Chopped

Dressing:

3 Tablespoons White Wine Vinegar

1 Teaspoon Dijon Mustard

1 Clove Garlic, Peeled & Chopped Fine

Direction:

In boiling water, drain the broccoli it on a paper towel.

Whisk together all dressing ingredients.

Toss ingredients together before serving.

great to cook with – extra virgin is best), many recommend taking a shot of cold oil olive daily! Bonus: if you don't like the taste or texture add a shot to your smoothie

Nutrition: Calories: 185, Protein: 4 g

Fat: 14 g, Carbs: 8 g

Interesting Facts: This oil is the main source of dietary fat in a variety of diets. It contains many vitamins and minerals that play a part in reducing the risk of stroke and lowers cholesterol and high blood pressure and can also aid in weight loss. It is best consumed cold, as when it is heated it can lose some of its nutritive properties (although it is still

28. Lentil Potato Salad

Servings: 2

Preparation Time: 35 Minutes

Ingredients:

½ Cup Beluga Lentils

8 Fingerling Potatoes

1 Cup Scallions, Sliced Thin

¼ Cup Cherry Tomatoes, Halved

¼ Cup Lemon Vinaigrette

Sea Salt & Black Pepper to Taste

Direction:

Bring two cups of water to simmer in a pot, adding your lentils. Cook for twenty to twenty-five minutes, and then drain. Your lentils should be tender.

Reduce to a simmer, cooking for fifteen minutes, and then drain. Halve your potatoes once they're cool enough to touch.

Put your lentils on a serving plate, and then top with scallions, potatoes, and tomatoes. Drizzle with your vinaigrette, and season with salt and pepper.

Nutrition: Calories: 400, Protein: 7 g

Fat: 26 g, Carbs: 39 g

Interesting Facts: Lemons are popularly known as harboring loads of Vitamin C, but are also excellent sources of folate, fiber, and antioxidants. Bonus: Helps lower cholesterol. Double Bonus: Reduces risk of cancer and high blood pressure.

29. Summer Chickpea Salad

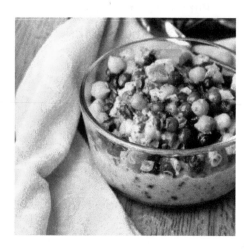

Servings: 4

Preparation Time: 15 Minutes

Ingredients:

1 ½ Cups Cherry Tomatoes, Halved

1 Cup English Cucumber, Slices

1 Cup Chickpeas, Canned, Unsalted, Drained & Rinsed

¼ Cup Red Onion, Slivered

2 Tablespoon Olive Oil

1 ½ Tablespoons Lemon Juice, Fresh

1 ½ Tablespoons Lemon Juice, Fresh

Sea Salt & Black Pepper to Taste

Direction:

Mix everything together and toss to combine before serving.

Nutrition: Calories: 145, Protein: 4 g, Fat: 7.5 g, Carbs: 16 g

30. Zucchini & Lemon Salad

Servings: 2

Preparation Time: 3 Hours 10 Minutes

Ingredients:

1 Green Zucchini, Sliced into Rounds

1 Yellow Squash, Zucchini, Sliced into Rounds

1 Clove Garlic, Peeled & Chopped

2 Tablespoons Olive Oil

2 Tablespoons Basil, Fresh

1 Lemon, Juiced & Zested

¼ Cup Coconut Milk

Sea Salt & Black Pepper to Taste

Direction:

Refrigerate all ingredients for three hours before serving.

Nutrition: Calories: 159, Protein: 3 g, Fat: 14 g, Net Carbs: 7 g

Interesting Facts: Lemons are popularly known as harboring loads of Vitamin C, but are also excellent sources of folate, fiber, and antioxidants. Bonus: Helps lower cholesterol. Double Bonus: Reduces risk of cancer and high blood pressure.

31. Watercress & Blood Orange Salad

Servings: 4

Preparation Time: 10 Minutes

Ingredients:

1 Tablespoon Hazelnuts, Toasted & Chopped

2 Blood Oranges (or Navel Oranges)

3 Cups watercress, Stems Removed

1/8 Teaspoon Sea Salt, Fine

1 Tablespoon Lemon Juice, Fresh

1 Tablespoon Honey, Raw

1 Tablespoon Water

2 Tablespoons Chives, Fresh

Direction:

Whisk your oil, honey, lemon juice, chives, salt and water together. Add in your watercress, tossing until it's coated.

Arrange the mixture onto salad plates, and top with orange slices. Drizzle with remaining liquid, and sprinkle with hazelnuts.

Nutrition: Calories: 94, Protein: 2 g, Fat: 5 g, Carbs: 13 g

Interesting Facts: Lemons are popularly known as harboring loads of Vitamin C, but are also excellent sources of folate, fiber, and antioxidants. Bonus: Helps lower cholesterol. Double Bonus: Reduces risk of cancer and high blood pressure.

32. Hearty Vegetarian Lasagna Soup

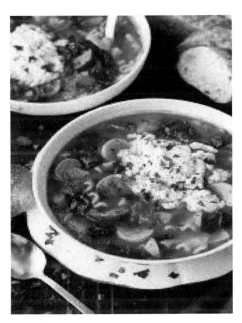

Servings: 10

Preparation time: 7 hours and 20 minutes

Ingredients:

12 ounces of lasagna noodles

4 cups of spinach leaves

2 cups of brown mushrooms, sliced

2 medium-sized zucchinis, stemmed and sliced

28 ounce of crushed tomatoes

1 medium-sized white onion, peeled and diced

2 teaspoon of minced garlic

1 tablespoon of dried basil

2 bay leaves

2 teaspoons of salt

1/8 teaspoon of red pepper flakes

2 teaspoons of ground black pepper

2 teaspoons of dried oregano

15-ounce of tomato sauce

6 cups of vegetable broth

Direction:

Grease a 6-quarts slow cooker and place all the ingredients in it except for the lasagna and spinach.

Cover the top, plug in the slow cooker; adjust the cooking time to 7 hours and let it cook on the low heat setting or until it is properly done.

In the meantime, cook the lasagna noodles in the boiling water for 7 to 10 minutes or until it gets soft.

Then drain and set it aside until the slow cooker is done cooking.

When it is done, add the lasagna noodles into the soup along with the spinach and continue cooking for 10 to 15 minutes or until the spinach leaves wilts.

Using a ladle, serving it in a bowl.

Nutrition: Calories:188 Cal, Carbohydrates:13g, Protein:18g, Fats:9g, Fiber:0g.

33. **Parsley Salad**

Servings: 8

Preparation Time: 30 Minutes

Ingredients:

3 Lemons, Juiced

150 g Flat Leaf Parsley, Chopped Fine

1 Cup Boiled Water

5 Tablespoons Olive Oil

Sea Salt & Black Pepper to Taste

6 Green Onions, Chopped Fine

1 Cup Bulgur

4 Tomatoes, Chopped Fine

Direction:

Add your Bulgur to your water and mix well. Put a towel on top of it to steam it. Keep it to the side, and then chop your spring onions, tomatoes and parsley. Put them in your salad bowl.

Pour your juice into the mixture, and then add in your olive oil, salt and pepper.

Put this mixture over your bulgur to serve.

Nutrition: Calories: 165.2, Protein: 3.8 g, Fat: 9.1 g, Carbs: 20.1 g

34. Tomato Eggplant Spinach Salad

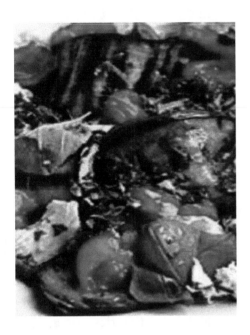

Preparation time: 30 minutes

Servings: 4

Ingredients:

1 large eggplant, cut into 3/4 inch slices

5 oz spinach

1 tbsp sun-dried tomatoes, chopped

1 tbsp oregano, chopped

1 tbsp parsley, chopped

1 tbsp fresh mint, chopped

1 tbsp shallot, chopped

For dressing:

1/4 cup olive oil

1/2 lemon juice

1/2 tsp smoked paprika

1 tsp Dijon mustard

1 tsp tahini

2 garlic cloves, minced

Pepper, *Salt*

Direction:

Place sliced eggplants into the large bowl and sprinkle with salt and set aside for minutes.

In a small bowl mix together all dressing ingredients. Set aside.

Heat grill to medium-high heat.

In a large bowl, add shallot, sun-dried tomatoes, herbs, and spinach.

Rinse eggplant slices and pat dry with paper towel.

Brush eggplant slices with olive oil and grill on medium high heat for 3-4 minutes on each side.

Let cool the grilled eggplant slices then cut into quarters. Add eggplant to the salad bowl and pour dressing over salad. Toss well.   Serve and enjoy.

 Nutrition: Calories: 163, Fat: 13 g, Carbohydrates: 10 g Sugar: 3 g, Protein 2 g

Cholesterol: 0 mg

35. Chunky Black Lentil Veggie Soup

Servings: 8

Preparation time: 4 hours and 35 minutes

Ingredients:

1 1/2 cups of black lentils, uncooked

2 small turnips, peeled and diced

10 medium-sized carrots, peeled and diced

1 medium-sized green bell pepper, cored and diced

3 cups of diced tomatoes

1 medium-sized white onion, peeled and diced

2 tablespoons of minced ginger

1 teaspoon of minced garlic

1 teaspoon of salt

1/2 teaspoon of ground coriander

1/2 teaspoon of ground cumin

3 tablespoons of unsalted butter

32 fluid ounce of vegetable broth

32 fluid ounce of water

Direction:

Using a medium-sized microwave, cover the bowl, place the lentils and pour in the water.

Microwave lentils for 10 minutes or until softened, stirring after 5 minutes.

Drain lentils and add to a 6-quarts slow cooker along with remaining ingredients and stir until just mix.

Cover with top, plug in slow cooker; adjust cooking time to 6 hours and let cook on low heat setting or until carrots are tender.   Serve straight away.

Nutrition: Calories: 90 Cal, Carbohydrates: 15g, Protein: 3g, Fats: 2g, Fiber: 3g.

36. Cauliflower Radish Salad

Preparation time: 15 minutes

Servings: 4

Ingredients:

12 radishes, trimmed and chopped

1 tsp dried dill

1 tsp Dijon mustard

1 tbsp cider vinegar

1 tbsp olive oil

1 cup parsley, chopped

½ medium cauliflower head, trimmed and chopped

½ tsp black pepper

¼ tsp sea salt

Direction:

In a mixing bowl, combine together cauliflower, parsley, and radishes.

In a small bowl, whisk together olive oil, dill, mustard, vinegar, pepper, and salt.

Pour dressing over salad and toss well.

Serve immediately and enjoy.

Nutrition: Calories: 58, Fat: 3.8 g, Carbohydrates: 5.6 g, Sugar: 2.1 g

Protein: 2.1 g, Cholesterol: 0 mg

37. **Celery Salad**

Preparation time: 10 minutes

Servings: 6

Ingredients:

6 cups celery, sliced

¼ tsp celery seed

1 tbsp lemon juice

2 tsp lemon zest, grated

1 tbsp parsley, chopped

1 tbsp olive oil

Sea salt

Direction:

Add all ingredients into the large mixing bowl and toss well.

Serve immediately and enjoy.

Nutrition: Calories: 38, Fat: 2.5g, Carbohydrates: 3.3 g, Sugar: 1.5g, Protein: 0.8g, Cholesterol 0 mg

38. <u>Citrus Salad</u>

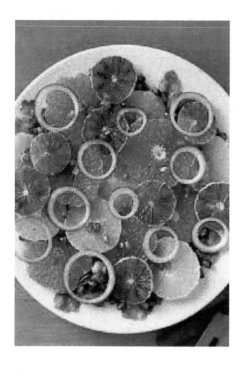

2 tbsp. honey

1 tbsp. shallot, minced

1 tbsp. fresh thyme, chopped

Salt and pepper to taste

4 cups mixed salad greens

2 cups radicchio leaves, shredded

3 oranges, sliced

1 grapefruit, sliced

¼ cup pomegranate seeds

Preparation Time: 10 Minutes

Cooking time: 0 minute

Servings: 8

Ingredients:

3 tbsp. freshly squeezed lemon juice

5 tbsp. olive oil

2 tsp. Dijon mustard

Direction:

Combine lemon juice, oil, mustard, honey, shallot, thyme, salt and pepper in a glass jar with lid.

Arrange the salad greens and radicchio leaves in a salad bowl.

Top with the oranges and grapefruit slices.

Sprinkle top with the pomegranate seeds.

Serve with the dressing on the side.

Nutrition:

Calories 144, Total Fat 9 g, Saturated Fat 1 g, Cholesterol 0 mg

Sodium 167 mg, Total Carbohydrate 16 g, Dietary Fiber 2 g

Protein 1 g, Total Sugars 12 g, Potassium 195 mg

39. Red Bell Pepper Salad

Preparation Time: 10 Minutes

Cooking time: 10 minutes

Servings: 4

Ingredients:

4 red bell peppers, sliced into quarters

4 oz. mozzarella cheese

3 tbsp. basil, chopped

1 tbsp. balsamic glaze

1 ½ tbsp. olive oil

Salt and pepper to taste

Direction:

Preheat your broiler.

Broil the bell peppers for 10 minutes.

Toss with the mozzarella and basil.

Drizzle with the balsamic glaze and olive oil.

Season with salt and pepper.

Nutrition:

Calories 166, Total Fat 13 g, Saturated Fat 5 g, Cholesterol 7 mg

Sodium 307mg, Total Carbohydrate 9g, Dietary Fiber 1g,

Protein6g, Total Sugars 5 g, Potassium 259 mg

40. **Spinach Salad**

Preparation Time: 10 Minutes

Cooking time: 0 minutes

Servings: 4

Ingredients:

2 tbsp. olive oil

Salt and pepper to taste

4 tsp. vinegar

8 cups baby spinach

1 cup raspberries

¼ cup goat cheese, crumbled

¼ cup hazelnuts, toasted and chopped

Direction:

Combine the vinegar, salt, pepper and oil in a bowl.

Toss the spinach and raspberries in this mixture.

Top with the goat cheese and hazelnuts.

Nutrition:

Calories 172, Total Fat 13 g, Saturated Fat 2 g, Cholesterol 3 mg

Sodium 267 mg, Total Carbohydrate 9 g, Dietary Fiber 5 g,

Protein 5 g, Total Sugars 2 g, Potassium 434 mg

41. Lovely Parsnip & Split Pea Soup

Servings: 8

Preparation time: 5 hours and 10 minutes

Ingredients:

1 tablespoon of olive oil

2 large parsnips, peeled and chopped

2 large carrots, peeled and chopped

1 medium-sized white onion, peeled and diced

1 1/2 teaspoon of minced garlic

2 1/4 cups of dried green split peas, rinsed

1 teaspoon of salt

1/2 teaspoon of ground black pepper

1 teaspoon of dried thyme

2 bay leaves

6 cups of vegetable broth

1 teaspoon of liquid smoke

Direction:

Place a medium-sized non-stick skillet pan over an average pressure of heat, add the oil and let it heat.

Add the parsnip, carrot, onion, garlic and let it cook for 5 minutes or until it is heated.

Transfer this mixture into a 6-quarts slow cooker and add the remaining ingredients.

Stir until mixes properly and cover the top.

Plug in the slow cooker; adjust the cooking time to 5 hours and let it cook on the high heat setting or until the peas and vegetables get soft.

When done, remove the bay leaf from the soup and blend it with a submersion blender or until the soup reaches your desired state.

Add the seasoning and serve.

Nutrition: Calories:199 Cal, Carbohydrates:21g, Protein:18g, Fats:5g, Fiber:8g.

42. Incredible Tomato Basil Soup

Servings: 6

Preparation time: 6 hours and 10 minutes

Ingredients:

1 cup of chopped celery

1 cup of chopped carrots

74 ounce of whole tomatoes, canned

2 cups of chopped white onion

2 teaspoons of minced garlic

1 tablespoon of salt

1/2 teaspoon of ground white pepper

1/4 cup of basil leaves and more for garnishing

1 bay leaf

32 fluid ounce of vegetable broth

1/2 cup of grated Parmesan cheese

Direction:

Using an 8 quarts or larger slow cooker, place all the ingredients.

Stir until it mixes properly and cover the top.

Plug in the slow cooker; adjust the cooking time to 5 hours and let it cook on the high heat setting or until the vegetables are tender. Blend the soup with a submersion blender or until soup reaches your desired state. Garnish it with the cheese, basil leaves and serve.

Nutrition: Calories:210 Cal, Carbohydrates: 11g, Protein: 12g, Fats: 10g, Fiber: 3g.

43. Chopped Cucumber, Tomato & Radish Salad

Preparation Time: 15 Minutes

Cooking time: 0 minute

Servings: 6

Ingredients:

1 tbsp. lemon juice

½ cup feta cheese, crumbled

½ cup mayonnaise

Salt and pepper to taste

1 tbsp. fresh dill, chopped

1 tbsp. fresh chives, chopped

1 cucumber, diced

3 cups cherry tomatoes, chopped

2 cups radish, diced

1 onion, minced

Direction:

Mix the lemon juice, feta cheese, mayo, salt, pepper, dill and chives in a bowl.

Stir in the rest of the ingredients.

Toss to coat evenly.

Nutrition: Calories 187, Total Fat 17 g, Saturated Fat 4 g, Cholesterol 0 mg, Sodium 40 mg, Total Carbohydrate 9 g, Dietary Fiber 2 g, Protein 10 g, Total Sugars 1 g, Potassium 164 mg

44. Spinach, Strawberry & Avocado Salad

Preparation Time: 5 Minutes

Cooking time: 0 minute

Servings: 2

Ingredients:

6 cups baby spinach

1 cup strawberries, sliced

2 tbsp. onion, chopped

½ avocado, diced

4 tbsp. vinaigrette

4 tbsp. walnuts, toasted

Direction:

Toss the spinach, strawberries, onion and avocado in the vinaigrette.

Sprinkle with the walnuts.

Nutrition:

Calories 296, Total Fat 18 g, Saturated Fat 2 g, Cholesterol 0 mg, Sodium 195 mg, Total Carbohydrate 27 g, Dietary Fiber 10 g, Protein 8 g, Total Sugars 11 g, Potassium 195 mg

45. Creamy Creamed Corn

Servings: 5

Preparation time: 4 hours

Ingredients:

16 ounce of frozen corn kernels

1 teaspoon of salt

1/2 teaspoon of ground black pepper

1 tablespoon honey

1/2 cup of vegetarian butter, unsalted

8-ounce of cream cheese, softened

1/2 cup of almond milk

Directions:

Take a 6-quarts slow cooker, grease it with a non-stick cooking spray and place ingredients in it.

Stir properly and cover the top.

Plug in the slow cooker; adjust the cooking time to 4 hours and let it cook on the low heat setting or until it is cooked thoroughly.

Serve right away.

Nutrition: Calories:120 Cal, Carbohydrates:28g, Protein:2g, Fats:1g, Fiber:4g.

46. Savory Squash & Apple Dish

Servings: 6

Preparation time: 4 hours and 15 minutes

Ingredients:

8 ounce of dried cranberries

4 medium-sized apples, peeled, cored and chopped

3 pounds of butternut squash, peeled, seeded and cubed

Half of a medium-sized white onion, peeled and diced

1 tablespoon of ground cinnamon

1 1/2 teaspoons of ground nutmeg

Directions:

Take a 6-quarts slow cooker, grease it with a non-stick cooking spray and place the ingredients in it.

Stir properly and cover the top.

Plug in the slow cooker; adjust the cooking time to 4 hours and let it cook on the low heat setting or until it cooks thoroughly.

Serve right away.

Nutrition: Calories:210 Cal, Carbohydrates:11g, Protein:3g, Fats:5g, Fiber:6g.

47. Spicy Cajun Boiled Peanuts

Servings: 15

Preparation time: 8 hours and 5 minutes

Ingredients:

5 pounds of peanuts, raw and in shells

6-ounce of dry crab boil

4-ounce of jalapeno peppers, sliced

2-ounce of vegetable broth

Directions:

Take a 6-quarts slow cooker place the ingredients in it and cover it with water.

Stir properly and cover the top.

Plug in the slow cooker; adjust the cooking time to 8 hours and let it cook on the low heat setting or until the peanuts are soft and floats on top of the cooking liquid.

Drain the nuts and serve right away.

Nutrition:

Calories:309 Cal, Carbohydrates: 5g, Protein: 0g, Fats: 26g, Fiber: 0g.

48. Wonderful Steamed Artichoke

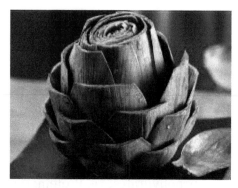

Servings: 4

Preparation time: 4 hours and 5 minutes

Ingredients:

8 medium-sized artichokes, stemmed and trimmed

2 teaspoons of salt

4 tablespoons of lemon juice

Directions:

Cut 1-inch part of the artichoke from the top and place it in a 6-quarts slow cooker, facing an upright position.

Using a bowl, place the lemon juice and pour in the salt until it mixes properly.

Pour this mixture over the artichoke and add the water to cover at least ¾ of the artichokes.

Cover the top, plug in the slow cooker; adjust the cooking time to 4 hours and let it cook on the high heat setting or until the artichokes get soft.

Serve immediately.

Nutrition: Calories: 78 Cal, Carbohydrates: 17g, Protein: 5g, Fats: 0g, Fiber: 9g.

49. Creamy Garlic Cauliflower Mashed Potatoes

Servings: 6

Preparation time: 3 hours

Ingredients:

30-ounce of cauliflower head, cut into florets

6 garlic cloves, peeled

1 teaspoon of salt

3/4 teaspoon of ground black pepper

1 bay leaf

1 tablespoon of vegetarian butter, unsalted

3 cups of water

Directions:

Take a 6-quarts slow cooker, grease it with a non-stick cooking spray and place the cauliflower florets into it.

Add the remaining ingredients except for the butter and stir properly. Cover the top, plug in the slow cooker; adjust the cooking time to 3 hours and let it cook on the high heat setting or until it is cooked thoroughly.

When done, open the slow cooker, remove the bay leaf and garlic cloves.

Drain the cooking liquid, add the butter and let it melt.

Then using an immersion blender, mash the cauliflower or until it gets creamy. Add the seasoning and serve.

Nutrition: Calories: 66 Cal, Carbohydrates: 6g, Protein: 3g, Fats: 4.2g, , Fiber: 3g.

50. Spicy Black Bean Burgers

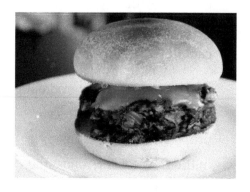

Preparation time: 25 min.

Servings: 6

Ingredients:

1 minced jalapeno pepper, small

1/2 cup flour

2 minced garlic cloves

1/2 tsp. oregano, dried

1 diced onion, small

1/2 cup corn niblets

2 cups mashed black beans, canned

1/4 cup breadcrumbs

2 tsp. minced parsley (optional)

1/4 tsp. cumin

1 tbsp. olive oil

1/2 diced red pepper, medium

2 tsp. chili powder

1/2 tsp. salt

Directions:

To coat, set aside the flour on a small plate. Sauté the garlic, onion, hot peppers, and oregano in oil on medium-high heat settings in a medium saucepan, until the onions are translucent. Put in the peppers & sauté until pepper is tender, approximately 2 more minutes. Keep it aside.

Use a fork or potato masher to mash the black beans in a large bowl. Stir in the vegetables cumin, breadcrumbs, chili powder, parsley, and salt. Mix well and divide to make 6 patties.

Coat each side of the patty by laying it down in the flour. Cook the patties on a lightly oiled frying pan until browned on either sides or approximately 10 minutes on medium-high heat.

Nutrition: 172.4 Calories, 3.2 g Total Fat, 0 mg Cholesterol, 29.7 g Total Carbohydrate, 7.1 g Dietary Fiber, 7.3 g Protein

51. Sushi Bowl

Servings: 1

Preparation Time: 40 Minutes

Ingredients:

½ Cup Edamame Beans, Shelled & Fresh

¾ Cup Brown Rice, Cooked

½ Cup Spinach, Chopped

¼ Cup Bell Pepper, Sliced

¼ Cup Avocado, Sliced

¼ Cup Cilantro, Fresh & Chopped

1 Scallion, Chopped

¼ Nori Sheet

1-2 Tablespoons Tamari

1 Tablespoon Sesame Seeds, Optional

Directions:

Steam your edamame beans, and then assemble your edamame, rice, avocado, spinach, cilantro, scallions and bell pepper into a bowl.

Cut the nori into ribbons, sprinkling it on top, drizzling with tamari and sesame seeds before serving.

Nutrition: Calories: 467, Protein: 22 g, Fat: 20 g, Carbs: 56 g

Interesting Facts: Avocados are known as miracle fruits in the world of Veganism. They are true super-fruit and incredibly beneficial. They are one of the best things to eat if you are looking to incorporate more fatty acids in your diet. They are also loaded with 20 various minerals and vitamins. Plus, they are easy to incorporate into dishes all throughout the day!

52. **Cauliflower Steaks**

Servings: 4

Preparation Time: 30 Minutes

Ingredients:

¼ Teaspoon Black Pepper

½ Teaspoon Sea Salt, Fine

1 Tablespoon Olive Oil

1 Head Cauliflower, Large

¼ Cup Creamy Hummus

2 Tablespoons Lemon Sauce

½ Cup Peanuts, Crushed
(Optional)

Directions:

Start by heating your oven to
425.

Cut your cauliflower stems,
and then remove the leaves.
Put the cut side down, and then
slice half down the middle. Cut
into ¾ inch steaks. If you cut

them thinner, they could fall
apart.

Arrange them in a single layer
on a baking sheet, drizzling
with oil. Season and bake for
twenty to twenty-five minutes.
They should be lightly browned
and tender.

Spread your hummus on the
steaks, drizzling with your
lemon sauce. Top with peanuts
if you're using it.

Nutrition: Calories: 167,
Protein: 6 g, Fat: 13 g, Carbs:
10 g

Interesting Facts: Cauliflower:
This vegetable is an extremely
high source of vitamin A,
vitamin B1, B2 and B3.

53. <u>Tofu Poke</u>

Servings: 4

Preparation Time: 30 Minutes

Calories: 262

Protein: 16 g

Fat: 15 g

Carbs: 19 g

Ingredients:

¾ Cup Scallions, Sliced Thin

1 ½ Tablespoons Mirin

¼ Cup Tamari

1 ½ Tablespoon Dark Sesame Oil, Toasted

1 Tablespoon Sesame Seeds, Toasted (Optional)

2 Teaspoons Ginger, fresh & Grated

½ Teaspoon Red Pepper, crushed

12 Ounces Extra Firm Tofu, Drained & Cut into ½ Inch Pieces

4 Cups Zucchini Noodles

2 Tablespoons Rice Vinegar

2 Cups Carrots, Shredded

2 Cups Pea Shoots

¼ Cup Basil, Fresh & Chopped

¼ Cup Peanuts, Toasted & Chopped (Optional)

Directions:

Whisk your tamari, mirin, sesame seeds, oil, ginger, red pepper, and scallion greens in a bowl. Set two tablespoons of this sauce aside and add the tofu to the remaining sauce. Toss to coat.

Combine your vinegar and zucchini noodles in a bowl.

Divide it between four bowls, topping with tofu, carrots, and a tablespoon of basil and peanuts.

Drizzle with sauce before serving.

Nutrition: Calories: 150, Protein: 8 g, Fat: 4 g, Carbs: 23 g

54. Tofu & Asparagus Stir Fry

Servings: 3

Preparation Time: 20 Minutes

Ingredients:

1 Tablespoon Ginger, Peeled & Grated

8 Ounces Firm Tofu, Chopped into Slices

4 Green Onions, Sliced Thin

Toasted Sesame Oil to Taste

1 Bunch Asparagus, Trimmed & Chopped

1 Handful Cashew Nuts, Chopped & Toasted

2 Tablespoons Hoisin Sauce

1 Lime, Juiced & Zested

1 Handful Mint, Fresh & Chopped

1 Handful Basil, Fresh & Chopped

3 Cloves Garlic, Chopped

3 Handfuls Spinach, Chopped

Pinch Sea Salt

Directions:

Get out a wok and heat up your oil. Add in your tofu, cooking for a few minutes.

Put your tofu to the side, and then sauté your red pepper flakes, ginger, salt, onions and asparagus for a minute.

Mix in your spinach, garlic, and cashews, cooking for another two minutes.

Add your tofu back in, and then drizzle in your lime juice, lime zest, hoisin sauce, cooking for another half a minute.

Remove it from heat, adding in your mint and basil.

Interesting Facts: Sesame seeds can be easily added to crackers, bread, salads, and stir-fry meals. Bonus: Help in lowering cholesterol and high blood pressure. Double bonus: Help with asthma, arthritis, and migraines!

Nutrition: Calories: 380, Protein: 22 g, Fat: 24 g, Carbs: 27 g

55. Edamame Salad

Servings: 1

Preparation Time: 15 Minutes

Ingredients:

¼ Cup Red Onion, Chopped

1 Cup Corn Kernels, Fresh

1 Cup Edamame Beans, Shelled & Thawed

1 Red Bell Pepper, Chopped

2-3 Tablespoons Lime Juice, Fresh

5-6 Basil Leaves, Fresh & Sliced

5-6 Mint Leaves, Fresh & Sliced

Sea Salt & Black Pepper to Taste

Direction:

Place everything into a Mason jar, and then seal the jar tightly. Shake well before serving.

Nutrition: Calories: 299, Protein: 20 g, Fat: 9 g, Carbs: 38 g

56. Fruity Kale Salad

Servings: 4

Preparation Time: 30 Minutes

Ingredients: Salad:

10 Ounces Baby Kale

½ Cup Pomegranate Arils

1 Tablespoon Olive Oil

1 Apple, Sliced

Dressing:

3 Tablespoons Apple Cider Vinegar

3 Tablespoons Olive Oil

1 Tablespoon Tahini Sauce (Optional)

Sea Salt & Black Pepper to Taste

Direction:

Wash and dry the kale. If kale is too expensive, you can also use lettuce, arugula or spinach. Take the stems out and chop it. Combine all your salad ingredients together. Combine all your dressing ingredients together before drizzling it over the salad to serve.

Nutrition: Calories: 220, Protein: 4 g, Fat: 17 g, Carbs: 16 g

57. Olive & Fennel Salad

Servings: 3

Preparation Time: 5 Minutes

Ingredients:

6 Tablespoons Olive Oil

3 Fennel Bulbs, Trimmed, Cored & Quartered

2 Tablespoons Parsley, Fresh & Chopped

1 Lemon, Juiced & Zested

12 Black Olives

Sea Salt & Black Pepper to Taste

Direction:

Grease your baking dish, and then place your fennel in it. Make sure the cut side is up. Mix your lemon zest, lemon juice, salt, pepper and oil, pouring it over your fennel. Sprinkle your olives over it and bake at 400.

Serve with parsley.

Nutrition: Calories: 331, Protein: 3 g, Fat: 29 g, Carbs: 15 g

58. Avocado & Radish Salad

Servings: 2

Preparation Time: 10 Minutes

Ingredients:

1 Avocado, Sliced

6 Radishes, Sliced

2 Tomatoes, Sliced

1 Lettuce Head, Leaves Separated

½ Red Onion, Peeled & Sliced

Dressing:

½ Cup Olive Oil

¼ Cup Lime Juice, Fresh

¼ Cup Apple Cider Vinegar

3 Cloves Garlic, Chopped Fine

Sea Salt & Black Pepper to Taste

Direction:

Spread your lettuce leaves on a platter, and then layer with your onion, tomatoes, avocado and radishes.

Whisk your dressing ingredients together before drizzling it over your salad.

Nutrition: Calories: 223, Protein: 3 g, Fat: 19 g, Carbs: 10 g

Interesting Facts: Avocados themselves are ranked within the top five of the healthiest foods on the planet, so you know that the oil that is produced from them is too. It is loaded with healthy fats and essential fatty acids. Like race bran oil it is perfect to cook with as well! Bonus: Helps in the prevention of diabetes and lowers cholesterol levels.

59. Black Bean & Corn Salad with Avocado

Servings: 6

Preparation time: 20 mins.

Ingredients:

1 and ½ cups corn kernels, cooked & frozen or canned

½ cup olive oil

1 minced clove garlic

⅓ cup lime juice, fresh

1 avocado (peeled, pitted & diced)

⅛ tsp. cayenne pepper

2 cans black beans, (approximately 15 oz.)

6 thinly sliced green onions

½ cup chopped cilantro, fresh

2 chopped tomatoes

1 chopped red bell pepper

Chili powder

½ tsp. salt

Direction:

In a small jar, place the olive oil, lime juice, garlic, cayenne, and salt.

Cover with lid; shake until all the ingredients under the jar are mixed well.

Toss the green onions, corn, beans, bell pepper, avocado, tomatoes, and cilantro together in a large bowl or plastic container with a cover. Shake the lime dressing for a second time and transfer it over the salad ingredients. Stir salad to coat the beans and vegetables with the dressing; cover & refrigerate. To blend the flavors completely, let this sit a moment or two. Remove the container from the refrigerator from time to time; turn upside down & back gently a couple of times to reorganize the dressing.

Nutrition: 448 Calories, 24.3 g Total Fat, 0 mg Cholesterol, 50.8 g Total

Carbohydrate, 14.3 g Dietary Fiber, 13.2 g Protein 30g

Chapter 7: Lunch and Dinner

60. Black Bean Burgers

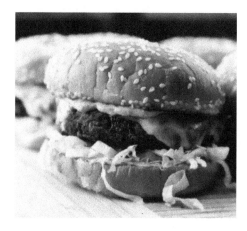

Servings: 6

Preparation Time: 25 Minutes

Ingredients:

1 Onion, Diced

½ Cup Corn Nibs

2 Cloves Garlic, Minced

½ Teaspoon Oregano, Dried

½ Cup Flour

1 Jalapeno Pepper, Small

2 Cups Black Beans, Mashed & Canned

¼ Cup Breadcrumbs (Vegan)

2 Teaspoons Parsley, Minced

¼ Teaspoon Cumin

1 Tablespoon Olive Oil

2 Teaspoons Chili Powder

½ Red Pepper, Diced

Sea Salt to Taste

Directions:

Set your flour on a plate, and then get out your garlic, onion, peppers and oregano, throwing it in a pan. Cook over medium-high heat, and then cook until the onions are translucent. Place the peppers in, and sauté until tender.

Cook for two minutes, and then set it to the side.

Use a potato masher to mash your black beans, and then stir

in the vegetables, cumin, breadcrumbs, parsley, salt and chili powder, and then divide it into six patties.

Coat each side, and then cook until it's fried on each side.

<u>Nutrition</u>: Calories: 173, Protein: 7.3 g, Fat: 3.2 g, Carbs: 29.7 g

Interesting Facts: Potatoes are a great starchy source of potassium and protein. They are pretty inexpensive if you are one that is watching their budget. Bonus: Very heart-healthy!

61. Dijon Maple Burgers

Servings: 12

Preparation Time: 50 Minutes

Ingredients:

1 Red Bell Pepper

19 Ounces Can Chickpeas, Rinsed & Drained

1 Cup Almonds, Ground

2 Teaspoons Dijon Mustard

1 Teaspoon Oregano

½ Teaspoon Sage

1 Cup Spinach, Fresh

1 – ½ Cups Rolled Oats

1 Clove Garlic, Pressed

½ Lemon, Juiced

2 Teaspoons Maple Syrup, Pure

Directions:

Get out a baking sheet. Line it with parchment paper.

Cut your red pepper in half and then take the seeds out. Place it on your baking sheet, and roast in the oven while you prepare your other ingredients. Process your chickpeas, almonds, mustard and maple syrup together in a food processor. Add in your lemon juice, oregano, sage, garlic and spinach, processing again. Make sure it's combined, but don't puree it.

Once your red bell pepper is softened, which should roughly take ten minutes, add this to the processor as well. Add in your oats, mixing well.

Form twelve patties, cooking in the oven for a half hour. They should be browned.

Nutrition: Calories: 200, Protein: 8 g, Fat: 11 g, Carbs: 21 g

Interesting Facts: Spinach is one of the most superb green veggies out there. Each serving is packed with 3 g of protein and is a highly encouraged component of the plant-based diet.

62. Hearty Black Lentil Curry

Servings: 4

Preparation time: 6 hours and 35 minutes

Ingredients:

1 cup of black lentils, rinsed and soaked overnight

14 ounce of chopped tomatoes

2 large white onions, peeled and sliced

1 1/2 teaspoon of minced garlic

1 teaspoon of grated ginger

1 red chili

1 teaspoon of salt

1/4 teaspoon of red chili powder

1 teaspoon of paprika

1 teaspoon of ground turmeric

2 teaspoons of ground cumin

2 teaspoons of ground coriander

1/2 cup of chopped coriander

4-ounce of vegetarian butter

4 fluid of ounce water

2 fluid of ounce vegetarian double cream

Directions:

Place a large pan over an average heat, add butter and let heat until melt.

Add the onion along with garlic and ginger and let cook for 10 to 15 minutes or until onions are caramelized.

Then stir in salt, red chili powder, paprika, turmeric, cumin, ground coriander, and water.

Transfer this mixture to a 6-quarts slow cooker and add tomatoes and red chili.

Drain lentils, add to slow
cooker and stir until just mix.

Plug in slow cooker; adjust
cooking time to 6 hours and let
cook on low heat setting.

When the lentils are done, stir
in cream and adjust the
seasoning.

Serve with boiled rice or whole
wheat bread.

Nutrition: Calories:527 Cal,
Carbohydrates:35g,
Protein:19g, Fats:34g, Fiber:6g.

63. Flavorful Refried Beans

Servings: 8

Preparation time: 8 hours and 15 minutes

Ingredients:

3 cups of pinto beans, rinsed

1 small jalapeno pepper, seeded and chopped

1 medium-sized white onion, peeled and sliced

2 tablespoons of minced garlic

5 teaspoons of salt

2 teaspoons of ground black pepper

1/4 teaspoon of ground cumin

9 cups of water

Directions:

Using a 6-quarts slow cooker, place all the ingredients and stir until it mixes properly.

Cover the top, plug in the slow cooker; adjust the cooking time to 6 hours, let it cook on high heat setting and add more water if the beans get too dry.

When the beans are done, drain them and reserve the liquid.

Mash the beans using a potato masher and pour in the reserved cooking liquid until it reaches your desired mixture.

Serve immediately.

Nutrition: Calories: 105 Cal, Carbohydrates: 36g, Protein: 13g, Fats: 1g, Fiber: 13g.

64. Spicy Black-Eyed Peas

Servings: 8

Preparation time: 8 hours and 20 minutes

Ingredients:

32-ounce black-eyed peas, un cooked

1 cup of chopped orange bell pepper

1 cup of chopped celery

8-ounce of chipotle peppers, chopped

1 cup of chopped carrot

1 cup of chopped white onion

1 teaspoon of minced garlic

3/4 teaspoon of salt

1/2 teaspoon of ground black pepper

2 teaspoons of liquid smoke flavoring

2 teaspoons of ground cumin

1 tablespoon of adobo sauce

2 tablespoons of olive oil

1 tablespoon of apple cider vinegar

4 cups of vegetable broth

Directions:

Place a medium-sized non-stick skillet pan over an average temperature of heat; add the bell peppers, carrot, onion, garlic, oil and vinegar.

Stir until it mixes properly and let it cook for 5 to 8 minutes or until it gets translucent.

Transfer this mixture to a 6-quarts slow cooker and add the peas, chipotle pepper, adobo sauce and the vegetable broth.

Stir until mixes properly and cover the top.

Plug in the slow cooker; adjust the cooking time to 8 hours and let it cook on the low heat setting or until peas are soft.

Serve right away.

Nutrition: Calories: 165 Cal, Carbohydrates: 23g, Protein: 6.7g, Fats: 2.5g, Fiber: 3.7g.

65. Exotic Butternut Squash and Chickpea Curry

Servings: 8

Preparation time: 6 hours and 15 minutes

Ingredients:

1 1/2 cups of shelled peas

1 1/2 cups of chickpeas, uncooked and rinsed

2 1/2 cups of diced butternut squash

12 ounce of chopped spinach

2 large tomatoes, diced

1 small white onion, peeled and chopped

1 teaspoon of minced garlic

1 teaspoon of salt

3 tablespoons of curry powder

14-ounce of coconut milk

3 cups of vegetable broth

1/4 cup of chopped cilantro

Directions:

Using a 6-quarts slow cooker, place all the ingredients into it except for the spinach and peas.

Cover the top, plug in the slow cooker; adjust the cooking time to 6 hours and let it cook on the high heat setting or until the chickpeas get tender.

30 minutes to ending your cooking, add the peas and spinach to the slow cooker and let it cook for the remaining 30 minutes.

Stir to check the sauce, if the sauce is runny, stir in a mixture of a tablespoon of cornstarch mixed with 2 tablespoons of water.

Serve with boiled rice.

Nutrition: Calories:243 Cal, Carbohydrates: 46g, Protein: 8g, Fats: 5.5g, Fiber: 11.6g.

66. Sizzling Vegetarian Fajitas

Servings: 8

Preparation time: 60 Minutes

Ingredients:

4 ounce of diced green chilies

3 medium-sized tomatoes, d iced

1 large green bell pepper, cored and sliced

1 large red bell pepper, cored and sliced

1 medium-sized white onion, peeled and sliced

1/2 teaspoon of garlic powder

1/4 teaspoon of salt

2 teaspoons of red chili powder

2 teaspoons of ground cumin

1/2 teaspoon of dried oregano

1 1/2 tablespoon of olive oil

Directions:

Take a 6-quarts slow cooker, grease it with a non-stick cooking spray and add all the ingredients. Stir until it mixes properly and cover the top.

Plug in the slow cooker; adjust the cooking time to 2 hours and let it cook on the high heat setting or until cooks thoroughly. Serve with tortillas.

Nutrition: Calories: 220 Cal, Carbohydrates: 73g, Protein: 12g, Fats: 8g, Fiber: 4g.

67. Rich Red Lentil Curry

Servings: 16

Preparation time: 8 hours and 10 minutes

Ingredients:

4 cups of brown lentils, uncooked and rinsed

2 medium-sized white onions, peeled and diced

2 teaspoons of minced garlic

1 tablespoon of minced ginger

1 teaspoon of salt

1/4 teaspoon of cayenne pepper

5 tablespoons of red curry paste

2 teaspoon of brown sugar

1 1/2 teaspoon of ground turmeric

1 tablespoon of garam masala

60-ounce of tomato puree

7 cups of water

1/2 cup of coconut milk

1/4 cup of chopped cilantro

Directions:

Using a 6-quarts slow cooker, place all the ingredients except for the coconut milk and cilantro.

Stir until it mixes properly and cover the top.

Plug in the slow cooker; adjust the cooking time to 5 hours and let it cook on the high heat setting or until the lentils are soft. Check the curry during cooking and add more water if needed.

When the curry is cooked, stir in the milk, then garnish it with the cilantro and serve right away.

Nutrition: Calories:192 Cal, Carbohydrates: 33g, Protein: 12g, Fats:3g, Fiber: 11g.

68. Exquisite Banana, Apple, and Coconut Curry

Servings: 6

Preparation time: 6 hours and 10 minutes

Ingredients:

1/2 cup of amaranth seeds

1 apple, cored and sliced

1 banana, sliced

1 1/2 cups of diced tomatoes

3 teaspoons of chopped parsley

1 green pepper, chopped

1 large white onion, peeled and diced

2 teaspoons of minced garlic

1 teaspoon of salt

1 teaspoon of ground cumin

2 1/2 tablespoons of curry powder

2 tablespoons of flour

2 bay leaves

1/2 cup of white wine

8 fluid ounce of coconut milk

1/2 cup of water

Directions:

Using a food processor place the apple, tomatoes, garlic and pulse it until it gets smooth but a little bit chunky. Add this mixture to a 6-quarts slow cooker and add the remaining ingredients. Stir until it mixes properly and cover the top.

Plug in the slow cooker; adjust the cooking time to 6 hours and let it cook on the low heat setting or until it is cooked thoroughly.

Add the seasoning and serve right away.

Nutrition: Calories:370 Cal, Carbohydrates: 15g, Protein: 5g, Fats: 8g, Fiber: 8g.

69. Tastiest Barbecued Tofu and Vegetables

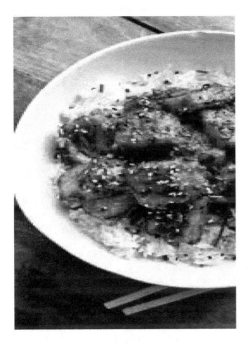

Servings: 4

Preparation time: 4 hours 15 minutes

Ingredients:

14-ounce of extra-firm tofu, pressed and drained

2 medium-sized zucchini, stemmed and diced

1/2 large green bell pepper, cored and cubed

3 stalks of broccoli stalks

8 ounce of sliced water chestnuts

1 small white onion, peeled and minced

1 1/2 teaspoon of minced garlic

2 teaspoons of minced ginger

1 1/2 teaspoon of salt

1/8 teaspoon of ground black pepper

1/4 teaspoon of crushed red pepper

1/4 teaspoon of five spice powder

2 teaspoons of molasses

1 tablespoon of whole-grain mustard

1/4 teaspoon of vegan Worcestershire sauce

8 ounces of tomato sauce

1/4 cup of hoisin sauce

1 tablespoon of soy sauce

2 tablespoons of apple cider vinegar

2 tablespoons of water

Directions:

Take a 6-quarts slow cooker, grease it with a non-stick cooking spray and set it aside until it is required.

Place a medium-sized non-stick skillet pan over an average heat, add the oil and let it heat.

Cut the tofu into 1/2 inch pieces and add it to the skillet pan in a single layer.

Cook for 3 minutes per sides and then transfer it to the prepared slow cooker.

When the tofu turns brown, place it into the pan, add the onion, garlic, ginger and cook for 3 to 5 minutes or until the onions are softened.

Add the remaining ingredients into the pan except for the vegetables which are the broccoli stalks, zucchini, bell pepper and water chestnuts.

Stir until it mixes properly and cook for 2 minutes or until the mixture starts bubbling.

Transfer this mixture into the slow cooker and stir properly.

Cover the top, plug in the slow cooker; adjust the cooking time to 3 hours and let it cook on the high heat setting or until it is cooked thoroughly.

In the meantime, trim the broccoli stalks and cut it into 1/4 inch pieces.

When the tofu is cooked thoroughly, put it into the slow cooker; add the broccoli stalks and the remaining vegetables.

Stir until it mixes properly and then return the top to cover it.

Continue cooking for 1 hour at the high heat setting or until the vegetables are tender.

Serve right away with rice.

Nutrition:

Calories:189 Cal,
Carbohydrates: 19g, Protein:
12g, Fats: 9g, Fiber: 3g.

70. Delightful Coconut Vegetarian Curry

Servings: 6

Preparation time: 4 hours and 20 minutes

Ingredients:

5 medium-sized potatoes, peeled and cut into 1-inch cubes

1/4 cup of curry powder

2 tablespoons of flour

1 tablespoon of chili powder

1/2 teaspoon of red pepper flakes

1/2 teaspoon of cayenne pepper

1 large green bell pepper, cut into strips

1 large red bell pepper, cut into strips

2 tablespoons of onion soup mix

14-ounce of coconut cream, unsweetened

3 cups of vegetable broth

2 medium-sized carrots, peeled and cut into matchstick

1 cup of green peas

1/4 cup of chopped cilantro

Directions:

Take a 6-quarts slow cooker, grease it with a non-stick cooking spray and place the potatoes pieces in the bottom.

Add the remaining ingredients except for the carrots, peas and cilantro.

Stir properly and cover the top.

Plug in the slow cooker; adjust the cooking time to 4 hours and let it cook on the low heat setting or until it cooks thoroughly.

When the cooking time is over, add the carrots to the curry and continue cooking for 30 minutes.

Then, add the peas and continue cooking for another 30 minutes or until the peas get tender.

Garnish it with cilantro and serve.

Nutrition: Calories: 369 Cal, Carbohydrates: 39g, Protein: 7g, Fats: 23g, Fiber: 8g

71. Super tasty Vegetarian Chili

Servings: 6

Preparation time: 2 hours and 10 minutes

Ingredients:

16-ounce of vegetarian baked beans

16 ounce of cooked chickpeas

16 ounce of cooked kidney beans

15 ounce of cooked corn

1 medium-sized green bell pepper, cored and chopped

2 stalks of celery, peeled and chopped

12 ounce of chopped tomatoes

1 medium-sized white onion, peeled and chopped

1 teaspoon of minced garlic

1 teaspoon of salt

1 tablespoon of red chili powder

1 tablespoon of dried oregano

1 tablespoon of dried basil

1 tablespoon of dried parsley

18-ounce of black bean soup

4-ounce of tomato puree

Directions:

Take a 6-quarts slow cooker, grease it with a non-stick cooking spray and place all the ingredients into it.

Stir properly and cover the top. Plug in the slow cooker; adjust the cooking time to 2 hours and let it cook on the high heat setting or until it is cooked thoroughly.

Serve right away.

Nutrition:

Calories: 190 Cal, Carbohydrates: 35g, Protein: 11g, Fats: 1g, Fiber: 10g

72. Creamy Sweet Potato & Coconut Curry

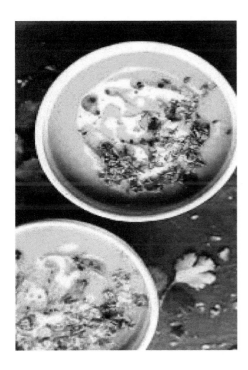

Servings: 6

Preparation time: 6 hours and 20 minutes

Ingredients:

2 pounds of sweet potatoes, peeled and chopped

1/2 pound of red cabbage, shredded

2 red chilies, seeded and sliced

2 medium-sized red bell peppers, cored and sliced

2 large white onions, peeled and sliced

1 1/2 teaspoon of minced garlic

1 teaspoon of grated ginger

1/2 teaspoon of salt

1 teaspoon of paprika

1/2 teaspoon of cayenne pepper

2 tablespoons of peanut butter

4 tablespoons of olive oil

12-ounce of tomato puree

14 fluid ounce of coconut milk

1/2 cup of chopped coriander

Directions:

Place a large non-stick skillet pan over an average heat, add 1 tablespoon of oil and let it heat. Then add the onion and cook for 10 minutes or until it

119

gets soft. Add the garlic, ginger, salt, paprika, cayenne pepper and continue cooking for 2 minutes or until it starts producing fragrance.

Transfer this mixture to a 6-quarts slow cooker and reserve the pan.

In the pan, add 1 tablespoon of oil and let it heat.

Add the cabbage, red chili, bell pepper and cook it for 5 minutes.

Then transfer this mixture to the slow cooker and reserve the pan.

Add the remaining oil to the pan; the sweet potatoes in a single layer and cook it in 3 batches for 5 minutes or until it starts getting brown.

Add the sweet potatoes to the slow cooker, along with tomato puree, coconut milk and stir properly. Cover the top, plug in the slow cooker; adjust the cooking time to 6 hours and let it cook on the low heat setting or until the sweet potatoes are tender. When done, add the seasoning and pour it in the peanut butter. Garnish it with coriander and serve.

Nutrition: Calories: 434 Cal, Carbohydrates: 47g, Protein: 6g, Fats: 22g, Fiber: 3g.

73. Comforting Chickpea Tagine

Servings: 6

Preparation time: 4 hours and 15 minutes

Ingredients:

14 ounce of cooked chickpeas

12 dried apricots

1 red bell pepper, cored and sliced

1 small butternut squash, peeled, cored and chopped

2 zucchini, stemmed and chopped

1 medium-sized white onion, peeled and chopped

1 teaspoon of minced garlic

1 teaspoon of ground ginger

1 1/2 teaspoon of salt

1 teaspoon of ground black pepper

1 teaspoon of ground cumin

2 teaspoon of paprika

1 teaspoon of harissa paste

2 teaspoon of honey

2 tablespoons of olive oil

1 pound of passata

1/4 cup of chopped coriander

Directions:

Take a 6-quarts slow cooker, grease it with a non-stick cooking spray and place the chickpeas, apricots, bell pepper, butternut squash, zucchini and onion into it.

Sprinkle it with salt, black pepper and set it aside until it is called for.

Place a large non-stick skillet pan over an average temperature of heat; add the oil, garlic, cumin and paprika.

Stir properly and cook for 1 minutes or until it starts producing fragrance.

Then pour in the harissa paste, honey, passata and boil the mixture.

When the mixture is done boiling, pour this mixture over the vegetables in the slow cooker and cover it with the lid.

Plug in the slow cooker; adjust the cooking time to 4 hours and let it cook on the high heat setting or until the vegetables gets tender.

When done, add the seasoning, garnish it with the coriander and serve right away.

Nutrition: Calories: 237 Cal, Carbohydrates: 45g, Protein: 9g, Fats: 2g, Fiber: 8g.

Chapter 8: Snacks and Desserts

74. Nori Snack Rolls

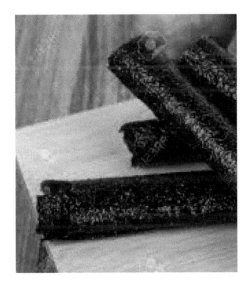

Preparation Time: 5 minutes

Cooking time: 10 minutes

Servings: 4 rolls

Ingredients

2 tablespoons almond, cashew, peanut, or others nut butter

2 tablespoons tamari, or soy sauce

4 standard nori sheets

1 mushroom, sliced

1 tablespoon pickled ginger

½ cup grated carrots

Directions:

Preparing the Ingredients.

Preheat the oven to 350°F.

Mix together the nut butter and tamari until smooth and very thick. Lay out a nori sheet, rough side up, the long way.

Spread a thin line of the tamari mixture on the far end of the nori sheet, from side to side. Lay the mushroom slices, ginger, and carrots in a line at the other end (the end closest to you).

Fold the vegetables inside the nori, rolling toward the tahini mixture, which will seal the roll. Repeat to make 4 rolls.

Put on a baking sheet and bake for 8 to 10 minutes, or until the rolls are slightly browned and crispy at the ends. Let the rolls cool for a few minutes, then slice each roll into 3 smaller pieces.

Nutrition (1 roll): Calories: 79; Total fat: 5g; Carbs: 6g; Fiber: 2g; Protein: 4g

75. Risotto Bites

Preparation Time: 15 minutes

Cooking time: 20 minutes

Servings: 12 bites

Ingredients

½ cup panko bread crumbs

1 teaspoon paprika

1 teaspoon chipotle powder or ground cayenne pepper

1½ cups cold Green Pea Risotto

Nonstick cooking spray

Directions:

Preparing the Ingredients.

Preheat the oven to 425°F.   Line a baking sheet with parchment paper.

On a large plate, combine the panko, paprika, and chipotle powder. Set aside.

Roll 2 tablespoons of the risotto into a ball.

Gently roll in the bread crumbs, and place on the prepared baking sheet. Repeat to make a total of 12 balls. Spritz the tops of the risotto bites with nonstick cooking spray and bake for 15 to 20 minutes, until they begin to brown. Cool completely before storing in a large airtight container in a single layer (add a piece of parchment paper for a second layer) or in a plastic freezer bag.

Nutrition (6 bites): Calories: 100; Fat: 2g; Protein: 6g; Carbohydrates: 17g; Fiber: 5g; Sugar: 2g; Sodium: 165

76. Tamari Toasted Almonds

Preparation Time: 2 minutes

Cooking time: 8 minutes

Servings: ½ cup

Ingredients

½ cup raw almonds, or sunflower seeds

2 tablespoons tamari, or soy sauce

1 teaspoon toasted sesame oil

Directions:

Preparing the Ingredients.

Heat a dry skillet to medium-high heat, then add the almonds, stirring very frequently to keep them from burning. Once the almonds are toasted, 7 to 8 minutes for almonds, or 3 to 4 minutes for sunflower seeds, pour the tamari and sesame oil into the hot skillet and stir to coat.

You can turn off the heat, and as the almonds cool the tamari mixture will stick to and dry on the nuts.

Nutrition (1 tablespoon): Calories: 89; Total fat: 8g; Carbs: 3g; Fiber: 2g; Protein: 4g

77. **Kale Chips**

Preparation Time: 5 minutes

Cooking time: 25 minutes

Servings: 2

Ingredients

1 large bunch kale

1 tablespoon extra-virgin olive oil

½ teaspoon chipotle powder

½ teaspoon smoked paprika

¼ teaspoon salt

Directions

Preparing the Ingredients.

Preheat the oven to 275°F.

Line a large baking sheet with parchment paper. In a large bowl, stem the kale and tear it into bite-size pieces. Add the olive oil, chipotle powder, smoked paprika, and salt.

Toss the kale with tongs or your hands, coating each piece well.

Spread the kale over the parchment paper in a single layer.

Bake for 25 minutes, turning halfway through, until crisp.

Cool for 10 to 15 minutes before dividing and storing in 2 airtight containers.

Nutrition: Calories: 144; Fat: 7g; Protein: 5g; Carbohydrates: 18g; Fiber: 3g;

Sugar: 0g; Sodium: 363mg

78. Savory Roasted Chickpeas

Preparation Time: 5 minutes

Cooking time: 25 minutes

Servings: 1 cup

Ingredients

1 (14-ounce) can chickpeas, rinsed and drained, or 1½ cups cooked

2 tablespoons tamari, or soy sauce

1 tablespoon nutritional yeast

1 teaspoon smoked paprika, or regular paprika

1 teaspoon onion powder

½ teaspoon garlic powder

Directions

Preparing the Ingredients.

Preheat the oven to 400°F.

Toss the chickpeas with all the other ingredients and spread them out on a baking sheet. Bake for 20 to 25 minutes, tossing halfway through.

Bake these at a lower temperature, until fully dried and crispy, if you want to keep them longer.

You can easily double the batch, and if you dry them out, they will keep about a week in an airtight container.

Nutrition (¼ cup) Calories: 121; Total fat: 2g; Carbs: 20g; Fiber: 6g; Protein: 8g

79. <u>Savory Seed Crackers</u>

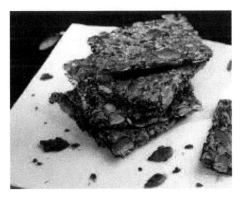

Preparation Time: 5 minutes

Cooking time: 50 minutes

Servings: 20 crackers

Ingredients

¾ cup pumpkin seeds
(pepitas)

½ cup sunflower seeds

½ cup sesame seeds

¼ cup chia seeds

1 teaspoon minced garlic
(about 1 clove)

1 teaspoon tamari or soy sauce

1 teaspoon vegan
Worcestershire sauce

½ teaspoon ground cayenne
pepper

½ teaspoon dried oregano

½ cup water

Directions

Preparing the Ingredients.

Preheat the oven to 325°F.

Line a rimmed baking sheet with parchment paper.

In a large bowl, combine the pumpkin seeds, sunflower seeds, sesame seeds, chia seeds, garlic, tamari, Worcestershire sauce, cayenne, oregano, and water.

Transfer to the prepared baking sheet, spreading out to all sides.

Bake for 25 minutes. Remove the pan from the oven and flip the seed "dough" over so the wet side is up. Bake for another 20 to 25 minutes, until the sides are browned.

Cool completely before breaking up into 20 pieces. Divide evenly among 4 glass jars and close tightly with lids.

Nutrition *(5 crackers):*

Calories: 339; Fat: 29g; Protein: 14g; Carbohydrates: 17g; Fiber: 8g; Sugar: 1g; Sodium: 96mg

80. Garlic Dip

Preparation time: 10 minutes

Cooking time: 0 minutes

Servings: 6

Ingredients:

1 cup coconut cream

4 garlic cloves, minced

2 tablespoons parsley, chopped

1 tablespoon lemon juice

Salt and black pepper to the taste

1 teaspoon garlic powder

1 tablespoon cilantro, chopped

Directions:

In a blender, combine the cream with the garlic, parsley and the other ingredients, pulse well, divide into small bowls and serve as a party dip.

Nutrition: calories 235, fat 12g, fiber 3g, carbs 6g, protein 1g

81. __Mushroom Bites__

Preparation time: 10 minutes

Cooking time: 20 minutes

Servings: 4

Ingredients:

1 pound baby Bella mushroom caps

1 teaspoon garlic powder

2 tablespoons olive oil

Salt and black pepper to the taste

1 teaspoon curry powder

1 tablespoon parsley, chopped

Directions:

In a bowl, mix the mushrooms with the oil, garlic powder and the other ingredients and toss well.

Spread the mushrooms on a baking sheet lined with parchment paper and cook in the oven at 350 degrees F for 20 minutes.

Arrange on a platter and serve as an appetizer.

Nutrition: calories 144, fat 20, fiber 3, carbs 7, protein 4g

82. **Coconut Spinach Balls**

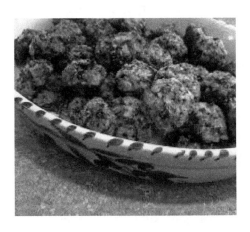

Preparation time: 10 minutes

Cooking time: 0 minutes

Servings: 12

Ingredients:

1 cup coconut cream

2 cups spinach, chopped

1 cup coconut, unsweetened and shredded

1 tablespoon psyllium powder

2 cups cashew cheese, grated

2 tablespoons Italian seasoning

Salt and black pepper to the taste

1 teaspoon parsley, dried

Directions:

In a bowl, mix the spinach with the cream and the other ingredients except the coconut and stir well.

Shape medium balls out of this mix, dredge them in coconut, arrange on a platter and serve.

Nutrition: calories 245, fat 12g, fiber 5g, carbs 3g, protein 4g

83. Zucchini Balls

Preparation time: 10 minutes

Cooking time: 8 minutes

Servings: 6

Ingredients:

2 tablespoons flaxseed mixed with 3 tablespoons water

1 pound zucchinis, grated

Salt and black pepper to the taste

¼ cup almond flour

1 cup cilantro, chopped

½ teaspoon garlic powder

2 tablespoons sun dried tomatoes, chopped

2 tablespoons olive oil

Directions:

in a bowl, mix the zucchinis with the flaxseed and the other ingredients except the oil, stir well and shape medium balls out of this mix.

Heat up a pan with the oil over medium high heat, drop the balls, cook them for 4 minutes on each side, drain excess grease on paper towels, arrange them on a platter and serve.

Nutrition: calories 80, fat 6, fiber 3, carbs 5, protein 7

84. Veggie Snack

Preparation time: 5 minutes

Cooking time: 20 minutes

Servings: 4

Ingredients:

1 cup cherry tomatoes, halved

1 cup radish, halved

1 cup black olives, pitted

2 tablespoons olive oil

1 teaspoon chili powder

Salt and black pepper to the taste

½ teaspoon Italian seasoning

A pinch of red pepper flakes, crushed

1 teaspoon garlic powder

Directions:

In a bowl, combine the tomatoes with the radishes and the other ingredients, toss, spread the veggies on a baking sheet lined with parchment paper and bake at 420 degrees F for 20 minutes.

Divide the veggies into bowls and serve as a snack.

Nutrition: calories 134, fat 8g, fiber 1g, carbs 0.5g, protein 8g

85. Nuts Balls

Preparation time: 10 minutes

Cooking time: 20 minutes

Servings: 12

Ingredients:

2 tablespoons flaxseed mixed with 3 tablespoons water

1 cup almonds, chopped

1 cup macadamia nuts, chopped

½ cup walnuts, chopped

1 cup coconut cream

¼ cup coconut, unsweetened and shredded

½ cup cashew cheese, grated

Salt and black pepper to the taste

1 tablespoon Italian seasoning

2 tablespoons coconut oil, melted

Cooking spray

Directions:

In a bowl, combine the flaxseed with the nuts, cream and the other ingredients except the cooking spray, whisk well and shape medium balls out of the mix. Arrange the balls on a baking sheet lined with parchment paper, grease with cooking spray and bake at 400 degrees F for 20 minutes.

Arrange the balls on a platter and serve.

Nutrition: calories 140, fat 5g, fiber 1g, carbs 3g, protein 4g

86. Berries Dip

Preparation time: 15 minutes

Cooking time: 0 minutes

Servings: 6

Ingredients:

1 cup blackberries

1 cup blueberries

1 cup coconut cream

1 teaspoon mint, dried

1 teaspoon stevia

Directions:

In a blender, combine the berries with the cream and the other ingredients, pulse well, divide into small bowls and keep in the fridge for 15 minutes before serving.

Nutrition: calories 150, fat 4g, fiber 0.4g, carbs 1.1g, protein 3g

87. **Cumin Olives Snack**

Preparation time: 10 minutes

Cooking time: 15 minutes

Servings: 4

Ingredients:

1 cup black olives, pitted

1 cup kalamata olives, pitted

½ cup cashew cheese, shredded

2 tablespoons avocado oil

Salt and black pepper to the taste

2 tablespoons cumin, ground

Directions:

In a bowl, combine the olives with the oil, cashew cheese and the other ingredients, toss well, spread them on a baking sheet lined with parchment paper and cook at 390 degrees F for 15 minutes. Divide the olives into bowls and serve as a snack.

Nutrition: calories 140, fat 6g, fiber 0, carbs 6g, protein 5g

88. Chives Fennel Salsa

Preparation time: 10 minutes

Cooking time: 0 minutes

Servings: 4

Ingredients:

2 fennel bulbs, shredded

½ cup chives, chopped

Juice of 1 lime

2 tablespoons olive oil

1 cup black olives, pitted and sliced

Salt and black pepper to the taste

2 celery stalks, finely chopped

2 tomatoes, cubed

Directions:

In a bowl, combine the fennel with the chives, lime juice and the other ingredients, toss well, divide into smaller bowls and serve as an appetizer.

Nutrition: calories 220, fat 7g, fiber 2, carbs 6g, protein 4g

89. <u>Hot Avocado Bites</u>

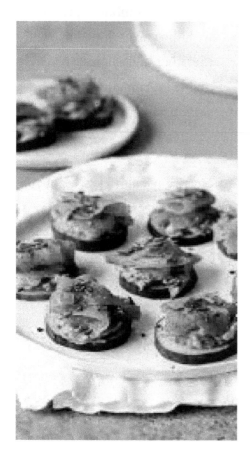

Preparation time: 5 minutes

Cooking time: 15 minutes

Servings: 4

Ingredients:

2 avocados, peeled, pitted and roughly cubed

2 tablespoons avocado oil

2 teaspoon chili powder

1 teaspoon sweet paprika

1 teaspoon rosemary, dried

Directions:

In a bowl, combine the avocados with the oil and the other ingredients, toss, spread them on a baking sheet lined with parchment paper and cook at 400 degrees F for 15 minutes.

Divide the avocado bites into bowls and serve as a snack.

<u>Nutrition</u>: calories 200, fat 16g, fiber 1, carbs 1g, protein 13g

90. Coffee Flavored Ice Cream

Servings:8

Preparation Time: 1 Hour And 30 Minutes

Ingredients:

1 cup unsweetened almond milk

2 1/2 cups heavy cream divided

1/2 cup powdered erythritol

1 tablespoon coconut oil

1/4 teaspoon xanthan gum

2 tablespoons instant coffee powder

1/2 teaspoon vanilla extract

1/4 teaspoon liquid stevia extract or to taste

Directions:

On medium fire, place a saucepan and mix a cup of heavy cream and almond milk.

Bring to a boil and then lower fire to a simmer. Frequently stirring, until reduced in half, around an hour and a half.

Turn off fire. Whisk in coconut oil ad erythritol until thoroughly combined and smooth. Whisk in liquid stevia extract, vanilla, coffee, and xanthan gum. Let it cool.

Meanwhile in a separate bowl, beat on high the remaining cream until stiff.

Once the coffee mixture is cooled, fold in whipped cream.

Transfer to a lidded container and freeze until solid.

Serve and enjoy.

Nutrition: Calories 150, Protein: 1g, Carbs: 2.5g, Sugar: 1g, Fat: 16g

91. Fudgy Almond Bars

Servings:8

Preparation Time: 10 Minutes

Ingredients:

1 cup almond flour

1 ounce dark chocolate or sugar-free chocolate chips

1/2 cup almond butter

1/2 cup unsalted butter (melted and divided)

1/2 teaspoon ground cinnamon

1/2 teaspoon vanilla extract

1/4 cup heavy cream

1/8 teaspoon xanthan gum

6 tablespoons powdered erythritol (divided)

Directions:

Line a 9x10-inch baking dish and preheat oven to 4000F.

In a medium mixing bowl, whisk well cinnamon, 2 tbsp powdered erythritol, ¼ cup melted butter, and almond flour.

Evenly spread mixture on bottom of prepared pan and pop in the oven. Bake until golden brown, around 10 minutes. Once done, remove from oven and cool completely.

In another mixing bowl, beat well 4 tbsp powdered erythritol, remaining butter, almond butter, and heavy cream. Stir in xanthan gum and vanilla. Mix well.

Evenly spread mixture on top of cooled crust. Sprinkle choco chips and refrigerate overnight.   Evenly slice into 8 bars and enjoy.

Nutrition: Calories 235, Protein: 4.5g, Carbs: 4g, Sugar: 2g Fat: 24g

92. Lava Cake Vegetarian Approved

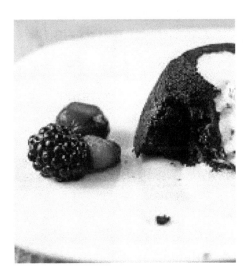

Servings:1

Preparation Time: 2 Minutes

Ingredients:

2 tbsp cocoa powder

1-2 tbsp erythritol

1 medium egg

1 tbsp heavy cream

1/2 tsp vanilla extract

1/4 tsp baking powder

1 pinch salt

Directions:

On a small mixing bowl, whisk well cocoa powder and erythritol.

In a different bowl, whisk egg until fluffy. Pour into bowl of cocoa and mix well.

Stir in vanilla and heavy cream mix well. Add baking powder and salt. Mix well.

Lightly grease a ramekin and pour in batter.

Stick in the microwave and cook for a minute on high. Let it rest for a minute. Serve and enjoy.

Nutrition: Calories 173, Protein: 8g, Carbs: 6g, Sugar: 2g Fat: 13g

93. Banana Pudding Approved

Servings:1

Preparation Time: 5 Minutes

Ingredients:

1 large egg yolk

1/2 cup heavy cream

1/2 tsp banana extract

1/2 tsp xanthan gum

3 tbsp powdered erythritol

Directions:

Place a large saucepan with 1-inch of water on medium high fire. Place a small pot inside the saucepan.

Add powdered erythritol, egg yolk, and heavy cream in small pot. Whisk well to mix and continue whisking until thickened.

Stir in xanthan gum and continue whisking to mix and thicken more.

Add salt and banana extract. Mix well.

Transfer to a small bowl and cover top completely with cling wrap.

Refrigerate for 4 hours and enjoy.

Nutrition:

Calories 455, Protein: 3g, Carbs: 5.5g, Sugar: 4.5g, Fat: 45g

94. Approved Mud Pie

Servings:10

Preparation Time: 40 Minutes

Ingredients:

1 ½ tsp baking soda

1 cup butter (melted)

1 cup erythritol

1/2 cup cocoa powder (sifted)

1/2 cup heavy cream

1/2 tsp salt

1/4 cup almond milk

2 cups almond flour

2 tbsp coconut flour

2 tsp vanilla extract

3 large eggs

Frosting Ingredients:

2 tbsp almond milk

1 1/2 tbsp cocoa powder

1/2 cup powdered erythritol

1/4 cup butter

Directions:

Lightly grease a 9x9-inch baking dish with cooking spray and preheat oven to 350oF.

In a mixing bowl, whisk well melted butter and eggs. Stir in heavy cream, baking soda, salt, almond milk, add vanilla extract, Mix thoroughly.

Add erythritol, cocoa powder, almond flour, and coconut flour. Mix well.

Pour into prepared dish and pop in the oven. Bake for 40 minutes and cool completely.

Meanwhile, make the frosting by melting butter in saucepan. Turn off fire and whisk in cocoa powder. Mix well.

Add almond milk and powdered erythritol and mix thoroughly until glossy and smooth.

Pour frosting on top of cake and refrigerate for at least an hour.

Slice into suggested and enjoy.

Nutrition: Calories: 400, Protein: 7g, Carbs: 6g, Sugar: 4g, Fat: 40g

95. Green Tea Mug Cake

Servings:1

Preparation Time: 12 Minutes

Ingredients:

1 large egg

1 tbsp coconut oil

1 tsp baking powder

1 pinch sea salt

2 tbsp frozen sugar-free white chocolate chips, frozen

½ tsp vanilla extract

½ tsp matcha powder

¼ cup almond flour

1/8 tsp xanthan gum

5-10 drops liquid stevia

1 ½ tbsp powdered erythritol

Directions:

Lightly grease the inside of a mug with cooking spray and preheat oven to 350oF.

In a small bowl, whisk well egg, coconut oil, baking powder, salt, vanilla, and liquid stevia. Stir in matcha powder, almond flour, xanthan gum, and erythritol. Mix well. Fold in frozen white choco chips. Transfer to prepared mug. Pop in the oven and bake for 12 minutes. Let cool a bit and enjoy.

Nutrition: Calories: 440, Protein: 14g, Carbs: 7g, Sugar: 5g, Fat: 38g

96. Chocolate Mousse with Avocado

Servings: 4

Preparation Time: 10 Minutes

Ingredients:

4 ounces chopped semisweet chocolate

2 large, ripe avocados

3 tablespoons unsweetened cocoa powder

1/4 cup Almond Breeze Unsweetened Almond Milk-Cashew milk Blend

1 teaspoon pure vanilla extract

1/8 teaspoon kosher salt

Directions:

In microwave safe bowl, place choco chips and microwave in 15-second interval while mixing every after microwaving until melted.

In food processor, add melted chocolate and remaining ingredients and puree until smooth and creamy.

Evenly divide into glasses and refrigerate for two hours before serving.

Nutrition: Calories per serving: 348, Protein: 6g, Carbs: 29g, Sugar: 14g, Fat: 27g

97. Brownie Muffin Approved

Servings:6

Preparation Time: 30 Minutes

Ingredients:

¼ cup cocoa powder

¼ cup slivered almonds

¼ cup sugar-free caramel syrup

½ cup pumpkin puree

½ tablespoon baking powder

½ teaspoon salt

1 cup golden flaxseed meal

1 large egg

1 tablespoon cinnamon

1 teaspoon apple cider vinegar

1 teaspoon vanilla extract

2 tablespoons coconut oil

Directions:

Line six muffin tins with muffin liners and preheat oven to 350oF.

In a large mixing bowl, whisk well egg and salt.

Whisk in caramel syrup, baking powder, pumpkin puree, cinnamon, apple cider, vanilla extract, and coconut oil. Mix thoroughly.

Add cocoa powder and flaxseed meal. Mix well.

Evenly divide batter into prepared muffin tins and sprinkle almonds on top.

Pop in the oven and bake for 15 minutes.

Cool and enjoy.

Nutrition: Calories per serving:193, Protein: 7g Carbs:11.5g, Sugar: 4.4g, Fat: 14g

98. **Brownies**

Servings: 6

Preparation Time: About 25 Minutes

Ingredients:

1 cup flaxseed meal

¼ cup cocoa powder

1 Tbsp. cinnamon

½ Tbsp. baking powder

½ tsp. salt

1 large egg

2 Tbsp. coconut oil

¼ cup sugar-free caramel syrup

½ cup pumpkin puree

1 tsp. vanilla extract

1 tsp. apple cider vinegar

¼ cup slivered almonds

Directions:

Preheat oven to 350 degrees Fahrenheit

Combine all the dry ingredients (flaxseed meal, cocoa powder, cinnamon, baking powder and salt) in aa large mixing bowl and whisk well to combine.

In a separate mixing bowl, combine the rest of the ingredients, excluding the almonds. Pour the wet ingredients into the dry ingredients and mix very well with a wooden spoon.

Put paper muffin liners in a muffin tin and spoon approximately ¼ cup of batter into each liner. Your Servings should be six muffins.

Sprinkle the almonds over the top of the batter, pressing them lightly into the surface so they stick.

Bake for about 15 minutes until the batter has risen and is set on top.

Nutrition: Total Fat: 14 g, Carbohydrates: 4 g, Protein: 7 g

Chapter 9: Smoothies and Drinks

99. Fruity Smoothie

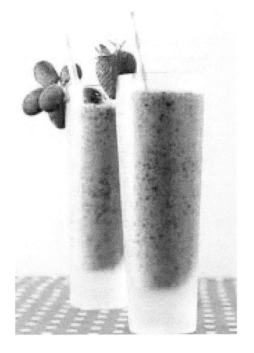

Preparation Time: 10 Minutes

Cooking time: 0 minute

Servings: 1

Ingredients:

¾ cup plain yogurt

½ cup pineapple juice

1 cup pineapple chunks

1 cup raspberries, sliced

1 cup blueberries, sliced

Direction:

Process the ingredients in a blender.

Chill before serving.

Nutrition: Calories 279, Total Fat 2 g, Saturated Fat 0 g

Cholesterol 4 mg, Sodium 149 mg, Total Carbohydrate 56 g

Dietary Fiber 7 g, Protein 12 g, Total Sugars 46 g, Potassium 719 mg.

100. Energizing Ginger Detox Tonic

Servings: 2

Preparation time: 15 minutes

Ingredients:

1/2 teaspoon of grated ginger, fresh

1 small lemon slice

1/8 teaspoon of cayenne pepper

1/8 teaspoon of ground turmeric

1/8 teaspoon of ground cinnamon

1 teaspoon of maple syrup

1 teaspoon of apple cider vinegar

2 cups of boiling water

Directions:

Pour the boiling water into a small saucepan, add and stir the ginger, then let it rest for 8 to 10 minutes, before covering the pan.

Pass the mixture through a strainer and into the liquid, add the cayenne pepper, turmeric, cinnamon and stir properly.

Add the maple syrup, vinegar, and lemon slice.

Add and stir an infused lemon and serve immediately.

Nutrition:

Calories:80 Cal, Carbohydrates: 0g, Protein: 0g, Fats: 0g, Fiber: 0g.

101. Warm Spiced Lemon Drink

Servings: 12

Preparation time: 2 hours and 10 minutes

Ingredients:

1 cinnamon stick, about 3 inches long

1/2 teaspoon of whole cloves

2 cups of coconut sugar

4 fluid of ounce pineapple juice

1/2 cup and 2 tablespoons of lemon juice

12 fluid ounce of orange juice

2 1/2 quarts of water

Directions:

Pour water into a 6-quarts slow cooker and stir the sugar and lemon juice properly.

Wrap the cinnamon, the whole cloves in cheesecloth and tie its corners with string.

Immerse this cheesecloth bag in the liquid present in the slow cooker and cover it with the lid.

Then plug in the slow cooker and let it cook on high heat setting for 2 hours or until it is heated thoroughly.

When done, discard the cheesecloth bag and serve the drink hot or cold.

Nutrition: Calories: 15 Cal, Carbohydrates: 3.2g, Protein: 0.1g, Fats: 0g, Fiber: 0g.

102. Soothing Ginger Tea Drink

Servings: 8

Preparation time: 2 hours and 15 minutes

Ingredients:

1 tablespoon of minced ginger root

2 tablespoons of honey

15 green tea bags

32 fluid ounce of white grape juice

2 quarts of boiling water

Directions:

Pour water into a 4-quarts slow cooker, immerse tea bags, cover the cooker and let stand for 10 minutes.

After 10 minutes, remove and discard tea bags and stir in remaining ingredients.

Return cover to slow cooker, then plug in and let cook at high heat setting for 2 hours or until heated through.

When done, strain the liquid and serve hot or cold.

Nutrition:

Calories:45 Cal, Carbohydrates:12g, Protein:0g, Fats:0g, Fiber:0g.

103. Nice Spiced Cherry Cider

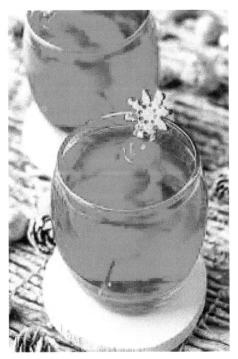

Servings: 16

Preparation time: 4 hours and 5 minutes

Ingredients:

2 cinnamon sticks, each about 3 inches long

6-ounce of cherry gelatin

4 quarts of apple cider

Directions:

Using a 6-quarts slow cooker, pour the apple cider and add the cinnamon stick.

Stir, then cover the slow cooker with its lid. Plug in the cooker and let it cook for 3 hours at the high heat setting or until it is heated thoroughly.

Then add and stir the gelatin properly, then continue cooking for another hour. When done, remove the cinnamon sticks and serve the drink hot or cold.

Nutrition: Calories: 100 Cal, Carbohydrates:0g, Protein:0g, Fats:0g, Fiber:0g

104.   Fragrant Spiced Coffee

Servings: 8

Preparation time: 2 hours and 10 minutes

Ingredients:

4 cinnamon sticks, each about 3 inches long

1 1/2 teaspoons of whole cloves

1/3 cup of honey

2-ounce of chocolate syrup

1/2 teaspoon of anise extract

8 cups of brewed coffee

Directions:

Pour the coffee in a 4-quarts slow cooker and pour in the remaining ingredients except for cinnamon and stir properly.

Wrap the whole cloves in cheesecloth and tie its corners with strings.

Immerse this cheesecloth bag in the liquid present in the slow cooker and cover it with the lid.

Then plug in the slow cooker and let it cook on the low heat setting for 3 hours or until heated thoroughly.

When done, discard the cheesecloth bag and serve.

Nutrition:

Calories:150 Cal, Carbohydrates:35g, Protein:3g, Fats:0g, Fiber:0g.

105. Tangy Spiced Cranberry Drink

Servings: 14

Preparation time: 2 hours and 10 minutes

Ingredients:

1 1/2 cups of coconut sugar

12 whole cloves

2 fluid ounce of lemon juice

6 fluid ounce of orange juice

32 fluid ounce of cranberry juice

8 cups of hot water

1/2 cup of Red Hot candies

Directions:

Pour the water into a 6-quarts slow cooker along with the cranberry juice, orange juice, and the lemon juice.

Stir the sugar properly.

Wrap the whole cloves in a cheese cloth, tie its corners with strings, and immerse it in the liquid present inside the slow cooker.

Add the red hot candies to the slow cooker and cover it with the lid.

Then plug in the slow cooker and let it cook on the low heat setting for 3 hours or until it is heated thoroughly.

When done, discard the cheesecloth bag and serve.

Nutrition: Calories:89 Cal, Carbohydrates:27g, Protein:0g, Fats:0g, Fiber:1g.

106. Warm Pomegranate Punch

Servings: 10

Preparation time: 2 hours and 15 minutes

Ingredients:

3 cinnamon sticks, each about 3 inches long

12 whole cloves

1/2 cup of coconut sugar

1/3 cup of lemon juice

32 fluid ounce of pomegranate juice

32 fluid ounce of apple juice, unsweetened

16 fluid ounce of brewed tea

Directions:

Using a 4-quart slow cooker, pour the lemon juice, pomegranate, juice apple juice, tea, and then sugar.

Wrap the whole cloves and cinnamon stick in a cheese cloth, tie its corners with a string, and immerse it in the liquid present in the slow cooker.

Then cover it with the lid, plug in the slow cooker and let it cook at the low heat setting for 3 hours or until it is heated thoroughly.

When done, discard the cheesecloth bag and serve it hot or cold.

Nutrition:

Calories:253 Cal, Carbohydrates:58g, Protein:7g, Fats:2g, Fiber:3g.

107. Rich Truffle Hot Chocolate

Servings: 4

Preparation time: 1 hours and 10 minutes

Ingredients:

1/3 cup of cocoa powder, unsweetened

1/3 cup of coconut sugar

1/8 teaspoon of salt

1/8 teaspoon of ground cinnamon

1 teaspoon of vanilla extract, unsweetened

32 fluid ounce of coconut milk

Directions:

Using a 2 quarts slow cooker, add all the ingredients and stir properly.

Cover it with the lid, then plug in the slow cooker and cook it for 2 hours on the high heat setting or until it is heated thoroughly.

When done, serve right away.

Nutrition: Calories:67 Cal, Carbohydrates:13g, Protein:2g, Fats:2g, Fiber:2.5g.

108. **Ultimate Mulled Wine**

Servings: 6

Preparation time: 35 minutes

Ingredients:

1 cup of cranberries, fresh

2 oranges, juiced

1 tablespoon of whole cloves

2 cinnamon sticks, each about 3 inches long

1 tablespoon of star anise

1/3 cup of honey

8 fluid ounce of apple cider

8 fluid ounce of cranberry juice

24 fluid ounce of red wine

Directions:

Using a 4 quarts slow cooker, add all the ingredients and stir properly. Cover it with the lid, then plug in the slow cooker and cook it for 30 minutes on the high heat setting or until it gets warm thoroughly.

When done, strain the wine and serve right away.

Nutrition: Calories:202 Cal, Carbohydrates:25g, Protein:0g, Fats:0g, Fiber:0g.

109. **Pleasant Lemonade**

Servings: 10 servings

Preparation time: 3 hours and 15 minutes

Ingredients:

Cinnamon sticks for serving

2 cups of coconut sugar

1/4 cup of honey

3 cups of lemon juice. fresh

32 fluid ounce of water

Directions:

Using a 4-quarts slow cooker, place all the ingredients except for the cinnamon sticks and stir properly.

Cover it with the lid, then plug in the slow cooker and cook it for 3 hours on the low heat setting or until it is heated thoroughly.

When done, stir properly and serve with the cinnamon sticks.

Nutrition:

Calories:146 Cal, Carbohydrates:34g, Protein:0g, Fats:0g, Fiber:0g.

110. **Pineapple, Banana & Spinach Smoothie**

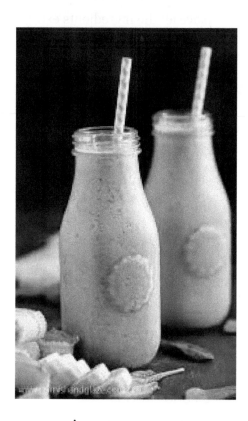

Preparation Time: 10 Minutes

Cooking time: 0 minute

Servings: 1

Ingredients:

½ cup almond milk

¼ cup yogurt

1 cup spinach

1 cup banana

1 cup pineapple chunks

1 tbsp. chia seeds

Direction:

Add all the ingredients in a blender.

Blend until smooth.

Chill in the refrigerator before serving.

Nutrition: Calories 297, Total Fat 6 g, Saturated Fat 1 g, Cholesterol 4 mg , Sodium 145 mg, Total Carbohydrate 54 g, Dietary Fiber 10 g Protein 13 g, Total Sugars 29g, Potassium 1038 mg

111. Kale & Avocado Smoothie

Preparation Time: 10 Minutes

Cooking time: 0 minute

Servings: 1

Ingredients:

1 ripe banana

1 cup kale

1 cup almond milk

¼ avocado

1 tbsp. chia seeds

2 tsp. honey

1 cup ice cubes

Direction:

Blend all the ingredients until smooth.

Nutrition: Calories 343, Total Fat 14 g, Saturated Fat 2 g

Cholesterol 0 mg, Sodium 199 mg, Total Carbohydrate 55 g

Dietary Fiber 12g, Protein 6g, Total Sugars 29g, Potassium 1051mg

112. Vegetable & Tomato Juice

Preparation Time: 10 Minutes

Cooking time: 0 minute

Servings: 2

Ingredients:

1 cup Romaine lettuce

¼ cup fresh chives, chopped

2 tomatoes, sliced

1 red bell pepper, sliced

2 stalks celery, chopped

1 carrot, chopped

Direction:

Process the ingredients in proper order using a juicer.

Pour the juice into glasses and serve.

Nutrition: Calories 46, Total Fat 0 g, Saturated Fat 0 g

Cholesterol 0 mg, Sodium 82 mg, Total Carbohydrate 9 g

Dietary Fiber 2 g, Protein 1g, Total Sugars 7 g, Potassium 466 mg

113. Orange & Carrot Juice

Nutrition:

Calories 111, Total Fat 1 g, Saturated Fat 0 g, Cholesterol 0 mg, Sodium 38 mg, Total Carbohydrate 24 g, Dietary Fiber 1g, Protein 2 g, Total Sugars 18 g,   Potassium 434 mg

Preparation Time: 15 Minutes

Cooking time: 0 minute

Servings: 2

Ingredients:

1 tomato, sliced

1 orange, sliced into wedges

1 apple, sliced

4 carrots, sliced

Ice cubes

Direction:

Follow the order of the ingredients list when processing these through the juice.

Transfer the juice into glasses.

Fill your glass with ice and serve.

114. Apple & Spinach Juice

Preparation Time: 10 Minutes

Cooking time: 0 minute

Servings: 2

Ingredients:

1½ cups spinach

½ grapefruit, sliced

2 apples, sliced

1 small ginger, sliced

2 stalks celery

Direction:

Process the ingredients in your juicer following the order in the list.

Pour juice into glasses and chill before serving.

Nutrition: Calories 55, Total Fat 0 g, Saturated Fat 0 g, Cholesterol 0 mg

Sodium 60 mg, Total Carbohydrate 13 g, Dietary Fiber 1 g, Protein 1 g, Total Sugars 10 g, Potassium 150 mg

115. Raspberry Chia Smoothie

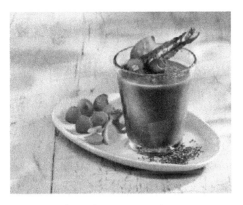

Preparation time: *30 Minutes*
Cooking time: 0 minutes
Servings: 01

Ingredients:

¾ cup of almond milk

1 cup raspberries

½ of a banana

1 tablespoon chia seeds

½ of an avocado

2 handful of spinach

Ice for thickness

Direction:

Add all the ingredients to a blender.

Hit the pulse button and blend till it is smooth.

Chill well and garnish as desired.

Serve.

Nutrition:

Calories 131, Total Fat 13 g, Saturated Fat 8g, Cholesterol 212 mg

Sodium 321mg, Total Carbs 9.7g, Fiber 3.1g, Sugar 1.8g, Protein2g

116. Banana Cinnamon Smoothie

Preparation time: *30 Minutes*
Cooking time: *0 minutes*
Servings: *01*

Ingredients:

1 cup unsweetened almond milk

½ cup oats

1 banana

1 tablespoon peanut butter

½ teaspoon cinnamon

A drizzle of maple syrup

Direction:

Add all the ingredients to a blender.

Hit the pulse button and blend till it is smooth.

Chill well to serve.

Nutrition: Calories 141, Total Fat 9 g, Saturated Fat 17g

Cholesterol 6 mg, Sodium 23 mg, Total Carbs 16 g, Fiber 4g

Sugar 3 g, Protein 3.1 g

117. Mango Carrot Smoothie

Preparation time: *30 Minutes*
Cooking time: *0 minutes*
Servings: *01*

Ingredients:

1 cup carrots, chopped

1 cup frozen mango

1 cup frozen pineapple

1 cup frozen strawberries

¼ cup soy yogurt

½ cup soy milk

1 tablespoon chia seeds

Direction:

Add all the ingredients to a blender.

Hit the pulse button and blend till it is smooth.

Chill well to serve.

Nutrition: Calories 64, Total Fat 0g, Saturated Fat 0g, Cholesterol 0 mg

Sodium 54 mg, Total Carbs 14.1 g, Sugar 0.3 g, Fiber 0.4 g, Protein 0.4 g

118. Green Glass Smoothie

Preparation time: *30 Minutes*
Cooking time: *0 minutes*
Servings: *01*

Ingredients:

1 cup baby spinach

½ cup cucumber, chopped

1 celery stalk

½ medium banana

½ cup pineapple

6 oz soy yogurt

¼ cup flax

½ cup of water

4 ice cubes

Direction:

Add all the ingredients to a blender.

Hit the pulse button and blend till it is smooth.

Chill well to serve.

Nutrition: Calories 61, Total Fat 1.3 g, Saturated Fat 0.7 g, Cholesterol 3 mg, Sodium 23 mg, Total Carbs 18.5 g, Sugar 11 g, Fiber 0.3 g, Protein 0.3

119. Blueberry Peach Tea Smoothie

Preparation time: *30 Minutes*
Cooking time: 0 minutes
Servings: 01

Ingredients:

1 cup black tea, brewed and cooled

5.3 ounces soy yogurt

1 cup blueberries

½ cup peaches

Ice

Direction:

Add all ingredients to a blender.

Hit the pulse button and blend till it is smooth.

Chill well to serve.

Nutrition:

Calories 19, Total Fat 0.4 g, Saturated Fat 0 g, Cholesterol 0 mg, Sodium 52 mg, Total Carbs 24.8 g, Sugar 2.4 g, Fiber 1.4 g, Protein 0.4 g

120. Beet Cinnamon Smoothie

Preparation time: *30 Minutes*
Cooking time: 0 minutes
Servings: 01

Ingredients:

2 cups almond milk

½ of a beet, cooked

3 tablespoons raw cacao powder

3-6 dates, pitted

½ teaspoon vanilla extract

¼ teaspoon ground cinnamon

1 pinch of salt

Direction:

Add all ingredients to a blender.

Hit the pulse button and blend till it is smooth.

Chill well to serve.

Nutrition: Calories 98, Total Fat 1.5 g, Saturated Fat 0 g, Cholesterol 0 mg, Sodium 94 mg, Total Carbs 31.5 g, Sugar 1.3 g, Fiber 0.1 g, Protein 10 g

121. MCT Green Smoothie

Preparation time: *30 Minutes*
Cooking time: 0 minutes
Servings: *01*

Ingredients:

1 ½ cups ice

1 banana

2 handfuls of spinach

½ avocado

2 cups almond milk

2 scoops plant-based protein powder

1 tablespoon MCT oil

Direction:

Add all ingredients to a blender.

Hit the pulse button and blend till it is smooth.

Chill well to serve.

Nutrition: Calories 121, Total Fat 1.2g, Saturated Fat 0.7g, Cholesterol 3 mg, Sodium 84 mg, Total Carbs 7.5 g, Sugar 6g Fiber 0.3 g, Protein 0.6 g

122. Pumpkin Fig Smoothie

Preparation time: *30 Minutes*
Cooking time: *0 minutes*
Servings: *01*

Ingredients:

½ large frozen banana

3 fresh figs

⅓ cup canned pumpkin

2 tablespoons almond butter

1 cup almond milk

3 ice cubes

1 tablespoon hemp hearts

Direction:

Add all ingredients to a blender.

Hit the pulse button and blend till it is smooth.

Chill well to serve.

Nutrition: Calories 115, Total Fat 1.1g, Saturated Fat 0.4 g, Cholesterol 2 mg,

Sodium 24 mg, Total Carbs 24.1 g, Sugar 1.3 g, Fiber 0.3 g, Protein 2.5 g

123. Orange Blueberry Blast

Preparation time: *30 Minutes*
Cooking time: *0 minutes*
Servings: *01*

Ingredients:

1 cup almond milk

1 scoop plant-based protein powder

1 cup blueberries

1 orange, peeled

1 teaspoon nutmeg

1 tablespoon shredded coconut

Direction:

Add all ingredients to a blender.

Hit the pulse button and blend till it is smooth.

Chill well to serve.

Nutrition:

Calories 185, Total Fat 0.1 g, Saturated Fat 0g, Cholesterol 0 mg, Sodium 144 mg, Total Carbs 6.1 g, Sugar 3.5 g, Fiber 0.1 g, Protein 0.1 g

124. Chocolate Peanut Butter Smoothie

Preparation time: *30 Minutes*
Cooking time: *0 minutes*
Servings: *01*

Ingredients:

1 cup almond milk

¼ cup quick oats

1 scoop plant-based protein powder

2 tablespoons peanut butter

2 teaspoons cocoa powder

1 tablespoon maple syrup

1 cup ice

Direction:

Add all ingredients to a blender.

Hit the pulse button and blend till it is smooth.

Chill well to serve.

Nutrition: Calories 109, Total Fat 12 g, Saturated Fat 03 g, Cholesterol 01 mg

Sodium 10 mg, Total Carbs 23.6 g, Sugar 2 g, Fiber 2.6 g, Protein 10 g

125. Miami Mango Shake

Preparation time: *30 Minutes*
Cooking time: *0 minutes*
Servings: *01*

Ingredients:

1 cup unsweetened coconut milk

1 scoop protein powder

1 cup frozen mango

1 cup frozen strawberries

Direction:

Add all ingredients to a blender.

Hit the pulse button and blend till it is smooth.

Chill well to serve.

Nutrition:

Calories 82, Total Fat 14 g, Saturated Fat 7 g, Cholesterol 632 mg

Sodium 497 mg, Total Carbs 6 g, Fiber 3 g Sugar 1 g, Protein 5 g

126. Hemp Green Smoothie

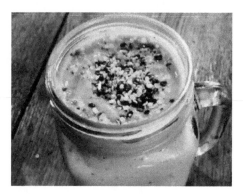

Preparation time: *30 Minutes*

Cooking time: 0 minutes

Servings: 01

Ingredients:

½ cup spinach

¼ avocado

½ banana, frozen

1 tablespoon hemp hearts

1 teaspoon chia seeds

1 cup almond milk

Direction:

Add all ingredients to a blender. Hit the pulse button and blend till it is smooth. Chill well to serve.

Nutrition: Calories 95, Total Fat 1.1 g, Saturated Fat 0.4 g, Cholesterol 2 mg, Sodium 84 mg, Total Carbs 2.1 g, Sugar 0.3 g, Fiber 0.6 g, Protein 2.4 g

127. **Infused water**

Preparation time: 5 Minutes

Cooking time: 20 minutes

Servings: 12

Ingredients:

1 lemon

1 orange

1 tbsp fresh ginger

5 cardamom pods

¼ tsp peppercorn

1 cinnamon stick

6 cups water

Directions:

Cut orange and lemon into slices and smash the cardamom pods. Peel the ginger and slice it up.

Add all ingredients to a pot and bring to a boil. Once boiling, stir and reduce the heat to a simmer. Let it simmer until the fruit slices break down.

Strain the liquid into a glass and serve with sugar if desired.

Nutrition: Calories 17, Sodium 4 mg, Total Carbs 4.3 g, Fiber 1.3 g, Sugar 1.6 g, Protein 0.5 g, Potassium 68 mg

128. Iced Tea

Preparation time: 5 Minutes

Cooking time: 0 minutes

Servings: 2

Ingredients:

A cup high quality tea bag

A tablespoon of coconut butter

A tablespoon of plant-based milk of your choice

Optional add-ins:

1 teaspoon of MCT oil

1 teaspoon of cinnamon

1 teaspoon of vanilla powder

1 teaspoon of coconut milk powder (instead of the plant milk)

Directions:

Brew your coffee – either a French press or automatic coffee maker using high-quality coffee.

Add a cup of coffee in a blender along with coconut butter and other add-ins and blend until foamy.

Pour in a mug and top with foamed plant milk or dust with cinnamon.

Nutrition: Calories 73, Total Fat 2.2 g, Saturated Fat 0.3 g, Cholesterol 1 mg, Sodium 9 mg, Total Carbs 11.7 g, Fiber 1.6 g, Sugar 6.2 g, Protein 2.3 g, Potassium 235 mg

Latte fantasy

Preparation time: 5 Minutes

Cooking time: 0 minutes

Servings: 2

Ingredients:

¼ cup almond or non-dairy milk

2 tbsp hemp seeds

Splash vanilla extract

1.5 frozen bananas, sliced into coins

Handful of ice

A few pinches cinnamon

1 cup cooled coffee (regular or decaf)

Directions:

Add the ice and keep blending on high until there are no lumps remaining. Taste for sweetness and add your preferred plant-based sugar or sugar alternative.

Transfer to a glass and serve.

Nutrition:

Calories 73, Total Fat 2.2 g, Saturated Fat 0.3 g, Cholesterol 1 mg, Sodium 9 mg, Total Carbs 11.7 g, Fiber 1.6 g, Sugar 6.2 g, Protein 2.3 g, Potassium 235 mg

130. **Chocolate**

Preparation time: 5 Minutes

Cooking time: 5 minutes

Servings: 2 cups

Ingredients:

3¼ cups almond milk

2/3 cups semi-sweet chocolate chips

1½ tsp ground cinnamon

1/8 tsp chili powder

1 tsp vanilla extract

pinch of cayenne pepper

Directions:

Add all ingredients to a saucepan and heat until chocolate melts.

Serve and enjoy.

Nutrition:

Calories 931, Total Fat 94.3 g, Saturated Fat 82.8 g, Cholesterol 0 mg, Sodium 77 mg, Total Carbs 26.4 g, Fiber 9.7 g, Sugar 15.3 g, Protein 9.2 g, Potassium 1,046 mg

131.   **Mocktail**

Preparation time: 15 Minutes

Preparation time: 15 Minutes

Cooking time: 10 minutes

Servings: 4

Ingredients:

¾ cup sugar

¾ cup water

1 package raspberries

1 sprig fresh mint

3 tbsp lime juice, freshly squeezed

6-8 oz sparkling mineral water

Crushed ice

Directions:

To make the basic syrup, add the sugar, water, and raspberries to a saucepan over medium heat. Mix occasionally until it starts to stew. Lower the heat and delicately stew it for 5 to 7 minutes.

Allow cooling then strain the syrup.

Muddle 3 to 4 tbsp of the syrup with 1 sprig of fresh mint at the bottom of the glass.

Add the lime juice, sparkling mineral water, and some crushed ice to the glass and stir.

Nutrition: Calories 145, Total Carbs 38.7 g, Fiber 0.3 g, Sugar 37.7 g, Protein 0.1 g, Potassium 27 mg

Chapter 10: Basic Shopping list

- eggs

- amaranth seeds

- apples

- banana

- tomatoes

- parsley

- Green pepper

- white onions

- garlic

- salt

- cumin

- curry powder

- flour

- bay leaves

- white wine

- coconut milk

- blueberries

- Green Zucchini

- kale

- extra-virgin olive oil

- chipotle powder

- paprika

- Olive Oil

- Basil

- Lemon

- Sea Salt

- Black Pepper

- maple syrup

- cinnamon

- baking powder

- baking soda

- unsweetened nut milk

- oats

- cashew butter

- vanilla plant-based protein powder

- buttermilk

- vanilla

- low-fat milk

- chives

- parsley

- black beans

- lentils

- carrot

- green bell peppers

- celery

- jalapeno pepper

- red onion

- apple cider vinegar

- brown rice

Chapter 11: 21 day meal plan

	BREAKFAT	LUNCH/DINNER	SNACKS/DESSERT
1.	Apple Pancakes	Sizzling Vegetarian Fajitas	Tomato and Basil Bruschetta
2.	Cream Cheese Waffles	Rich Red Lentil Curry	Savory Roasted Chickpeas
3.	Herb & Cheese Omelet	Exotic Butternut Squash and Chickpea Curry	Avocado and Tempeh Bacon Wraps
4.	Pineapple Bagel with Cream Cheese	Spicy Black-Eyed Peas	Tamari Toasted Almonds
5.	Scrambled Eggs with Spinach	Flavorful Refried Beans	Garden Salad Wraps
6.	Oatmeal Pancake	Smoky Red Beans and Rice	Curried Tofu "Egg Salad" Pitas
7.	Waffles with Pumpkin & Cream Cheese	Hearty Black Lentil Curry	Jicama and Guacamole
8.	Avocado & Egg Salad on Toasted Bread	Dijon Maple Burgers	Risotto Bites
9.	Cottage Cheese, Honey & Raspberries	Black Bean Burgers	Nori Snack Rolls

10.	Apple Pancakes	Savory Spanish Rice Comforting Chickpea Tagine	Burgers
11.	Cream Cheese Waffles	Creamy Sweet Potato & Coconut Curry	Brownie Muffin Approved
12.	Herb & Cheese Omelet	Super tasty Vegetarian Chili	Chocolate Mousse with Avocado
13.	Pineapple Bagel with Cream Cheese	Delightful Coconut Vegetarian Curry	Green Tea Mug Cake
14.	Scrambled Eggs with Spinach	Tastiest Barbecued Tofu and Vegetables	Approved Mud Pie
15.	Oatmeal Pancake	Exquisite Banana, Apple, and Coconut Curry	Lava Cake Vegetarian Approved
16.	Waffles with Pumpkin & Cream Cheese	Sizzling Vegetarian Fajitas	Banana Pudding Approved
17.	Avocado & Egg Salad on Toasted Bread	Rich Red Lentil Curry	Coffee Flavored Ice Cream
18.	Cottage Cheese, Honey & Raspberries	Exotic Butternut Squash and Chickpea Curry	Fudgy Almond Bars

19.	Apple Pancakes	Spicy Black-Eyed Peas	Chives Fennel Salsa
20.	Cream Cheese Waffles	Flavorful Refried Beans	Hot Avocado Bites
21.	Herb & Cheese Omelet	Smoky Red Beans and Rice	Berries Dip

Conclusion

Without commitment, it will be impossible for you to achieve your set goals. Develop a practical plan that will help you transition smoothly into the plant-based lifestyle. While doing this, you should make sure that your environment is conducive to allowing you to focus on your diet plan. Your efforts should be directed towards learning more about the plant-only diet. For instance, you should subscribe to YouTube channels where you can watch and enjoy videos of other vegans as they delve into their experiences. When making a leap from other diets to plant-based diets, anything can happen along the way. Of course, there are instances where you might fall off the wagon and turn to animal-based diets or processed foods. However, what you should know is that it is normal to fall and regress once in a while. The transformation is not easy; therefore, forgive yourself for making mistakes here and there. Focus on the bigger picture of living a blissful life where you are at a lower risk of cancer, diabetes, and other ailments. More importantly, keep yourself inspired by connecting with like-minded people. Don't overlook their importance in the transition, as they are also going through the challenge you are facing. Hence, they should advise you from time to time on what to do when you feel stuck.

All the best!

PLANT BASED HIGH PROTEIN COOKBOOK

Introduction

You will be amazed by the benefits that eating whole foods can bring you. Within weeks, you may notice that you have more energy and feel greater than ever. On top of the added benefit of health, you will also be helping the environment and the animals. As you will soon be learning in the following chapters, fruits and vegetables do not need to be bland! You will be provided with dozens of delicious recipes for breakfast, lunch, and dinner.

Whether you are seasoned in the kitchen or a true beginner, this book was created for any individual who wishes to add vegan meals into their diet so that they can experience the incredible health results. All recipes that you find within this book are plant-based meals, which were created to celebrate the natural and rich flavors of your fruits and vegetables. You will find that the foods provide the nutritional value you need, which can help you fight disease and lose weight. Once you have a clear understanding of a Vegan diet, you will be learning all about high-protein foods that you will be consuming. There are many myths behind the vegan diet such as lack of nutrients and vitamins now that you will no longer be consuming animal products. The truth is nature provides us with everything we need! When you feel confident with the rules of the diet, then it is time to get to the fun action: cooking!

I hope that by the end of this book, you will be inspired to create the flavorful and protein-packed meals provided within this chapter. Each recipe is quick, easy-to-follow, and packed with the vitamins and nutrients that you need to maintain a healthy balance through breakfast, lunch, and dinner. I have assured to include a wide variety of recipes to appease even the skeptical carnivore in your life. The recipes in this book are simple to make and will inspire you to keep going. But you need not limit yourself to just these ideas. Feel free to come up with some recipes of your own. As long as you make use of the core ingredients, you can experiment to your heart's content! Let's begin!

Chapter 1: What is protein?

Healthy protein is thought to be the foundation of life, considering that it is in every cell of the body.

Healthy protein is composed of amino acids that are connected to each other in lengthy chains. There are 20 different types of amino acids, and the series in which the various amino acids are set up aids to establish the duty of that specific healthy protein.

Healthy proteins contribute to:

- Transferring particles throughout the body.
- Assisting the repair service of cells and making brand-new ones.
- Safeguarding the body from germs and infections.

- Provide appropriate development and growth in youngsters, young adults, and expectant females.

Without loading your diet plan with the proper quantities of healthy protein, you risk losing out on those crucial features. At some point, that can bring troubles, such as a loss of muscular tissue mass, that failing to expand, compromise the performance of the heart and lungs - leading to death.

One of the most shared and well-known structures in our body that rely on protein is our muscles. Muscles are attached to the bone, thus allowing us to move and function daily. While this is most obvious, the organs in our body use internal muscles to make sure that we are working and ensuring every part is doing exactly what it was intended to. Even though several parts of our body are not made of protein, they tend to be held together by protein. This includes our nervous system, organs, and blood vessels. This should show you why protein is so important in our diet.

Without a diet that contains proper protein nutrition, you would lack the components needed for tissue repair, protein to support enzymes and hormones for metabolic functions, and the aid to antibodies that help in the defense against germs and infections. While all of this may scare you away from the vegan diet or to over-consume protein, don't do this. I say this for several reasons...

For one, if you want to follow a vegan diet, I am actually going to show you that it is very possible, with all the recipes in this book! Second, if you go crazy and overload protein into your body, this can, in fact, affect your body in negative ways. Yes, there are issues if you don't have the needed amount, and yes there are issues if you take too much protein into your system. Finding the right healthy protein balance is an important thing to keep in mind when living the vegan lifestyle.

The Importance of Protein in Your Diet

Protein is a macronutrient and a very important constituent of a diet whether   you are looking to build muscle or not, as:

- It is a constituent of all body cells. As a matter of fact, nails and hair are mostly made of protein.

- Protein is required to repair and build tissue.
- Hormones, enzymes, and many other important body chemicals are made up of protein.
- It is a vital building block of cartilage, muscles, bones, skin, and blood.
- Our bodies do not stock up on protein like they do carbohydrates and fats, hence it has no reserve to draw from when the dietary requirement is not being met.

Chapter 2: Protein Requirement and How to Calculate Protein RDA Best for your Body

Healthy protein is a vital nutrient; its intake is essential for the wellness of your muscle mass and, for the wellness of the heart. Consuming healthy protein can, also, aid you handle specific illness and sustain your weight-loss initiatives. The quantity of healthy protein you need to take in is based upon your weight, exercise, age and various other variables.

Computing the RDA for protein

To figure out just how much healthy protein you ought to be consuming, there is a simple formula: take your weight, which you most likely recognize in extra pounds, and then you need to transform it to kgs. The ordinary American male evaluates to have 195.7 extra pounds (matching approximately 88.77 kilos), while the typical American woman evaluates to have 168.5 extra pounds (which amounts to a concerning 75.21 kilos).

Considering that most individuals need to consume about 0.8 grams of healthy protein per kilo of body weight, this implies that the RDA formula is:

(0.8 grams of healthy protein) x (weight in kilos).

Provided this standard, many males should consider that they should have an intake of 71 grams of healthy protein daily, due to the fact that 0.8 x 88.77 = 71.016. Ladies should eat around 60 grams of healthy protein each day, considering that the equation gives 0.8 x 75.21 = 60.168.

You can additionally simply increase your weight in extra pounds by 0.36 grams of healthy protein if you are having problem computing your body weight in kilos. This would change the RDA formula to the following:

(0.36 grams of healthy protein) x (weight in extra pounds).

There is a selection of healthy protein consumption calculators offered online if you are not comfortable in computing your RDA for healthy protein by hand. You can use sites like the "United States Department of Agriculture's Dietary Reference Intakes Calculator".

Individuals who need more protein

The RDA for healthy protein usually is 0.8 gram per kilo of body weight, lots of individuals can take in extra healthy protein safely. Professional athletes, for example, can eat as much of healthy protein as they desire as they burn a lot by exercising. Other individuals, like expecting females, nursing mothers and older generations additionally require eating even more of this nutrient.

The quantity of healthy protein you ought to eat as a professional athlete relies on the sort of exercise you take part in. Generally, individuals carrying out different workout routines ought to eat:

Minimum exercise (periodic stroll or extending): 1.0 gram

of healthy protein per kilo of body weight.

Modest exercise (regular weight-lifting, quick strolling): 1.3 grams of healthy protein per kg of body weight.

Extreme training (professional athletes, routine joggers): 1.6 grams of healthy protein per kilo of body weight.

Expectant ladies, likewise, require eating even more healthy protein than the standard suggested. According to a 2016 research in the Journal of Advances in Nutrition, women need to take in between 1.2 and 1.52 grams of healthy protein per kilo of weight every day while pregnant.

The reduced quantity (1.2 grams) is appropriate for very early maternities stages of around 16 weeks, while the top quantity is advised for later maternities of about 36 weeks.

The assumption of healthy protein by expectant ladies isn't just crucial for the development of the fetus; it is additionally vital in assisting the mother's body prepare to nurse their kids.

How to calculate your protein needs

It is crucial that we consume a sufficient amount of healthy protein each day to cover our body's requirements. Do you recognize just how much healthy protein you require?

Numerous professional athletes and other people that work out a lot assume that they ought to enhance their healthy protein consumption to assist them to shed their weight or construct even more muscle mass. It is real that the extra you work out, the higher your healthy protein requirement will undoubtedly be.

Healthy protein intake guidelines

Healthy proteins are the standard foundation of the body. They are comprised of amino acids and are required for the formation of muscular tissues, blood, skin, hair, nails, and the wellbeing of the interior body's organs. Besides water, healthy protein is one of the most abundant compounds in the body, and the majority of it is in the skeletal muscle mass.

Considering this, it is assuring to understand that according to the Dietary Guidelines for Americans between 2015-2020, most individuals obtain sufficient healthy protein daily. The very same record directs out that the consumption of fish and shellfish, and plant-based proteins such as seeds and nuts, are frequently lacking.

If you are an athlete, nonetheless, your healthy protein requirements might be somewhat greater considering that resistance training and endurance exercises can swiftly break down muscular tissue healthy protein.

If you are attempting to gain even more muscular tissue, you might assume that you require a lot healthier protein, yet this is not what you should do. There is proof that very strict professional athletes or exercisers might take in even more healthy protein (over 3 grams/kilograms daily), but for the typical exerciser, consumption of as much as 2 grams/per kg daily suffices for building muscle mass.

Various ways to determine protein needs

When establishing your healthy protein requirements,

you can either recognize a percent of overall day-to-day calories, or you can target in detail the number of grams of healthy protein to eat each day.

Percent of daily calories

Present USDA nutritional standards recommend that adult males and females should take an amount in between 10 and 35 percent of their overall calories intake from healthy protein. To obtain your number and to track your consumption, you'll require to understand the number of calories you eat daily.

To keep a healthy and balanced weight, you need to take in about the same variety of calories that you burn daily.

Just increase that number by 10 percent and by 35 percent to obtain your variety when you understand precisely how many calories you take in daily.

As an example, a male that eats 2,000 calories each day would require to eat between 200 to 700 calories every day of healthy protein.

Healthy protein grams each day

As an option to the portion method, you can target the specific amount of healthy protein grams each day.

One straightforward method to obtain an amount of healthy protein grams daily is to equate the percent array into a particular healthy protein gram variety. The mathematical formula for this is very easy.

Each gram of healthy protein consists of 4 calories, so you will just need to split both calorie array numbers by 4.

A guy that consumes 2,000 calories daily must take in between 200 and 700 calories from healthy protein or 50 to 175 grams of healthy protein.

There are various other methods to obtain a much more specific number which might consider lean muscular tissue mass and/or exercise degree.

You can establish your fundamental healthy protein requirement as a percent of your complete day-to-day calorie consumption or as a series of healthy protein grams daily.

Healthy protein needs based on weight and activity

The ordinary adult demands a minimum of 0.8 grams of healthy protein per kg of body weight each day. One kg equates to 2.2 extra pounds, so an individual that has 165 extra pounds or 75 kg would require

around 60 grams of healthy protein daily.

Healthy protein needs based on lean body mass

A new approach of finding out how much healthy protein you require is focused on the degree of the exercise (how much energy you spend) and your lean body mass. Some professionals really feel that this is an exact extra method because our lean body mass needs extra healthy protein for upkeep than fat.

Lean body mass (LBM) is merely the quantity of bodyweight that is not fat. There are various methods to identify your lean body mass, yet the most convenient is to deduct your body fat from your overall body mass.

You'll require to establish your body fat percent. There are various methods to obtain the number of your body fat consisting of screening with skin calipers, BIA ranges, or DEXA scans. You can approximate your body fat with the following calculating formula.

To determine your overall body fat in extra pounds, you will need to increase your body weight by the body fat portion. If you evaluate yourself to be 150 pounds and that your fat percent is 30, then 45 of those bodyweight pounds would certainly be fat (150 x 30% = 45).

Compute lean body mass. Merely deduct your body fat weight from your overall body weight. Utilizing the exact same instance, the lean body mass would certainly be 105 (150 - 45 = 105).

Calculating your protein needs

While the above standards offer you a general idea of where your healthy protein consumption needs to drop, determining the quantity of day-to-day healthy protein that's right for you, there is another method that can assist you in tweaking the previous results.

To identify your healthy protein requirements in grams (g), you need to initially determine your weight in kgs (kg) by separating your weight in pounds by 2.2.

Next off, choose the number of grams of healthy protein per kilo of bodyweight that is appropriate for you.

Use the reduced end of the array (0.8 g per kg) if you consider yourself to be healthy but not very active.

You should intake a more significant amount of protein (in between 1.2 and 2.0) if you are under tension, expecting, recuperating from a health problem, or if you are associated with extreme and constant weight or endurance training.

(You might require the recommendations of a physician or nutritional expert to assist you to establish this number).

Increase your weight in kg times the number of healthy protein grams per day.

For instance:

A 154 pound man that has as a routine exercising and lifting weights, but is not training at an elite degree:

154 lb/2.2 = 70 kg.

70 kg x 1.7 = 119 grams healthy protein each day.

Healthy protein as a percent of complete calories

An additional means to determine how much healthy protein you require is utilizing your everyday calorie consumption and the percentage of calories that will certainly originate from healthy protein.

Figure out exactly how many calories your body requires each day to keep your current weight.

Discover what your basal metabolic rate (BMR) is by utilizing a BMR calculator (often described as a basic power expense, or BEE, calculator).

Figure out the amount of calories you burn via day-to-day tasks and include that number to your BMR.

Next off, choose what portion of your diet plan will certainly originate from healthy protein. The percent you pick will certainly be based upon your objectives, physical fitness degree, age, type of body, and your metabolic rate. The Dietary Guidelines for Americans 2015-2020 advises that healthy protein represent something in between 10 percent and 35 percent for grownups suggested caloric intake.

Multiply that percentage by the complete variety of calories your body requires for the day to establish overall everyday calories from healthy protein.

Split that number by 4. (Quick Reference - 4 calories = 1 gram of healthy protein.)

For instance:

A 140-pound woman that eats 1800 calories each day consuming a diet plan having 20 percent of the total caloric intake consisting of healthy protein:

1800 x 0.20 = 360 calories from healthy protein.

360 calories/ 4 = 90 grams of healthy protein each day.

Compute daily protein need

To establish your day-to-day healthy protein requirement, increase your LBM by the suitable task degree.

Less active (normally non-active): increase by 0.5.

Light task (consists of strolling or horticulture): increase by 0.6.

Modest (30 mins of a modest task, thrice weekly): increase by 0.7.

Energetic (one hour of workout, 5 times regular): increase by 0.8.

Really energetic (10 to 20 hrs of regular workout): increase by 0.9.

Professional athlete (over 20 hrs of regular workout): increase by 1.0.

Based upon this approach, a 150-pound individual with an LBM of 105 would certainly need a day-to-day healthy protein amount that varies between 53 grams (if inactive) to 120 grams (if very active).

How many grams of protein should you eat per kilogram of body weight?

The quantity of healthy protein you take in is essential for your wellness. Lots of people ought to take in 0.8 grams of healthy protein per kilo of body weight, however, this quantity can alter based upon different elements. Individuals that are expecting, lactating, that have particular health and wellness problems or that are extremely energetic, commonly need even more healthy protein than the standard.

Healthy protein requirement per kilogram

You need to recognize your healthy protein demand per kg of body weight. Basically, the Recommended Dietary Allowance or RDA for healthy protein is 0.8 gram per kg of body weight.

Specific diet plans, like low-carbohydrate diet plans or the Atkins diet and even paleo diet regimens, might need you to eat even more healthy protein than this while still permitting you to take in a well-balanced diet regimen. Various other diet plans, like the Dukan diet or the predator diet regimen, concentrate on consuming only healthy protein and fat.

Raising the quantity of healthy protein you consume can be healthy and balanced and excellent, mainly if the healthy protein you are eating is originating from different resources. However, according to the Harvard Medical School, taking in even more than 2 grams of healthy protein per kg of body weight or even more can be harmful to your wellness.

According to the Centers for Disease Control, the ordinary American male values 195.7 extra pounds (or 88.77 kilos), while the typical American lady values 168.5 extra pounds (or 75.21 kilos). Given that the RDA is 0.8 grams of healthy protein for every single kilo of body weight, this indicates that a lot of males need to take in about 71 grams of healthy protein daily. Females that are a bit smaller sized ought to generally take in around 60 grams of healthy protein each day.

Chapter 3: Macros and Micronutrient

Macronutrients or macros and micronutrients or micros are molecules that the human body needs to survive, properly function and avoid getting ill. We need macros in large amounts as they are the primary nutrients for our body. There are three main macronutrients: carbohydrates, proteins, and fats. Micronutrients such as vitamins, minerals, and electrolytes are the other type of nutrients that human body requires, but in comparison to macros, micros are required in much smaller amounts.

Except for fad diets, the human body needs all three macronutrients and cutting out any of the macronutrients puts the risk of nutrient deficiencies and illness on human health.

Carbohydrates that you eat is a source of quick energy, they are transformed into glucose or commonly known as sugar and are either used right after generated or stored as glycogen for later use.

Protein is there to help with growth, injury repair, muscle formation, and protection against infections. Proteins are the compounds that are built from amino acids, which appear to be the building material for the creation of tissues in the human body. And our body needs 20 various amino acids, 9 of which cannot be produced by our body, and thus must be received from outside sources.

Dietary fat is another essential macronutrient that is responsible for many essential tasks like absorbing the fat-soluble vitamins (A, D, E and K), insulating body during cold weather, surviving long periods without food, protecting organs, supporting cell growth, and inducing hormone production.

Usually, to stay healthy, lose weight and for some other reasons we are told to count the number of calories that we intake entirely, forgetting to tell to track macronutrient intake. Calculating and monitoring macronutrient intake can help not only with making health better and reaching fitness goals but can also help you understand which types of foods improve your performance and which are bad for you. If you would like to get such a calculator, you can type in a Google search, and there you will get lots of information on the topic.

You have most likely listened to many talks about macros if you have been in the health and fitness environment for any length of time. Comprehending the truths behind macros and concerning your individual dietary needs will certainly make a difference in your very own wellness journey. In this chapter, we'll discover what macros are, exactly how to recognize if you are consuming the appropriate proportions and the very best foods for supplying them.

Macronutrients are the food classifications that give you the power to bring out our fundamental human features, and they are boiled down right into 3 groups: healthy protein, fats, and carbs. When you recognize precisely how to determine your macros, it is simple to figure out just how much calories you are placing in your body every day and just how much energy you require to burn off the extra calories.

The 3 macronutrients are carbs, fats, and healthy proteins, and they all have various duties in your body. Generally, you'll drop weight. If you desire to obtain an insight into how to monitor your macros, then keep reading.

Carbohydrates:

Composed of starches and sugars, carbohydrates are the macronutrient that your system most calls for. Your body breaks down a lot of carbs as soon as they are ingested, so they are accountable for providing you with an essential source of energy. Unless you get on a specialized consuming strategy like the ketogenic diet plan, carbohydrates ought to compose roughly 45-65% of your caloric requirements.

Carbs provide your body with sugar, its key energy source. When sugar goes into a cell, a collection of metabolic responses transforms it right into ATP (Adenosine Triphosphate), which is a kind of temporary power. Any extra sugar is changed right into a starch called glycogen, which is saved in the liver and as body fat for later usage.

Not all carbs are developed equivalent, as not all carbs are quickly absorbable or can be used for power manufacturing. Cellulose, as an example, is a non-digestible carb found in vegetables and fruits that serves as a nutritional fiber. This indicates that it aids the body get rid of waste from the big intestinal tract, subsequently maintaining it in functioning order.

Much shorter particles are much easier for your body to break down, so they are identified as basic. Complicated carbohydrates, in comparison, are bigger particles that your body takes longer to break down. Despite these distinctions, a carbohydrate is a carbohydrate in concerns to your macros.

Healthy protein:

All healthy proteins are made up of mixes of twenty various amino acids, which your body subsequently damages apart and incorporates to develop various physical structures. In other words, your body requires healthy protein to sustain the body's organ performance, power enzyme responses, and to construct your hair, nails, and various other cells.

Of the twenty amino acids, 9 are categorized as necessary, implying that your body cannot produce them, so you require to take them in via food. Those that consume a plant-based diet regimen rather than following an omnivorous diet can likewise satisfy their amino acid requirements by consuming a healthy diet plan that is composed of numerous plant-based resources of healthy protein like nuts, vegetables, and entire grains.

Like carbs, one gram of healthy protein includes 4 calories.

Fat:

Despite their destructive credibility in previous years, you should not outlaw fats from your diet plan. Your body requires fats to remain healthy and balanced, and in between 10-35% of your food needs to be composed of this macronutrient.

Fats additionally work as a power source, as it is your

body's recommended approach for saving extra calories. Your system will just keep percentages of sugar in your cells, yet body fat allows you safe and secure unrestricted amounts of power rather, which you use while resting, throughout the workout, and in between meals.

When you start consuming fats, you are required to guarantee that you provide your system with fats it needs, and that cannot make itself, like omega-3 and omega-6 fats. You can find omega-3s in oily fish, eggs and walnuts, and omega-6s from a lot of veggie oils.

Water

Water makes up a considerable part of our bodies. It manages our body temperature level and helps in the metabolic process.

The Institute of Medicine suggests drinking 13 cups of water (about 3 liters) for males and 9 cups (or 2.2 liters) for females. Not sure if you are getting enough water?

Just how to figure out your macronutrient requirements

While nutritional experts advise particular proportions of each macronutrient for ideal health and wellness, every person's dietary demands will certainly be various. You can identify your specific macronutrient levels with these actions.

1. Identify your calorie requirements:

Your day-to-day calorie requirements depend on lots of variables, including your age, weight, physical fitness level, and a lot more. You can establish your degrees by tracking what you consume in an ordinary week (one in which you aren't shedding or getting weight). The ordinary degree from nowadays is an excellent indication of your calorie requirements.

2. Transform calorie counts to macronutrients

You can designate these calories in the direction of macronutrients based on the proportion you are following when you understand your calorie targets. Frequently, the macronutrient intakes varies between (AMDR) 45-65% of your day-to-day calories from carbohydrates, 20-35% from fats, and 10-35% from healthy protein.

Next off, you can identify the variety of grams to you readily available with standard mathematics. Right, here's an instance:

By thinking you require 2,000 calories daily, you can establish your fat consumption by increasing 2,000 by 0.20 (the proportion of fat for 40:40:20 macronutrient divides). That completes 400, which is the variety of daily calories to dedicate to nutritional fat. To establish your gram consumption, divide 400 by 9 (the calories in a gram of fat) for a complete need of 44 grams of fat daily.

Tips for tracking your macronutrients

Are you prepared to begin checking your macro levels? One vital action is identifying which foods will certainly aid you to achieve your goals. Eat your carbohydrates, healthy protein, and fat, so if you stick to eating those, you will make sure you are optimizing your macros.

When you initially begin checking macros, it is ideal to utilize a food range to distribute the grams amount. After you are comfortable eyeballing the quantities, you can place the food straight on your plate.

Following your body's macronutrient requirements is a clever method to remain in control of your health and wellness. The procedure of tracking grams of food could appear challenging, yet with this method, you'll acquire the abilities needed to make sure each dish is healthy enough to enhance your health and wellness.

Why do individuals count macros?

While we might be used to counting calories, a macro-focused diet plan isn't about the number of calories in your food, instead what sort of calories they are.

"To be healthy and balanced, it is crucial to obtain the best equilibrium of macros in your diet regimen," Dr. Ali states. "Sometimes individuals likewise count macros if they're attempting to drop weight, or for various other factors, such as if they're attempting to ensure they obtain the correct amount of healthy protein they require to get muscular tissue".

Locating that equilibrium suggests recognizing specifically what your body demands and what you intend to acquire or shed. It needs some computations; however, the advantages can be significant.

If It Fits Your Macros (IIFYM) diet regimen merely implies making use of a macro calculator to maintain track of the percent of healthy protein, fats, and the carbohydrates you are consuming.

Is there a fundamental macro calculator anybody can utilize?

Yes ... yet it will undoubtedly need some mathematics.

You require to figure out your basal metabolic rate or BMR. This is the rate at which your body utilizes the energy consumed and differs from one person to another. There are on the internet calculators to aid you with this, or you can do the formula on your own.

For females aged 18-30 it is: 0.0546 x (weight in kilos) + 2.33

For those aged 30-60 it is: 0.0407 x (weight in kilos) + 2.90

You can, after that, use your overall energy expense for a day.

If you are much less energetic than the basic population you increase it by 1.49 if you are at an ordinary level, you increase it by 1.63, and if you are much more energetic you increase it by 1.78

That's the amount of calories you require each day. Still with me?

From here, you can determine your macro beginning factor. Dr. Ali describes: "As a wide estimation, healthy proteins, and carbs, offer us 4 calories for each gram, and fat offers us 9 grams. If you consume a tiny smoked chicken breast, which has 6.4 g of fat and 29g of healthy protein, it would undoubtedly have 58 calories from fat and 116 calories from healthy protein - so 174 calories overall".

"We require around 50% of our calories from carbs, 15% from healthy protein, and 35% from fat, nevertheless, this obviously changes for different people".

"Regardless of whether you are attempting to slim down or construct muscular tissue, you maintain the percentages of 50% carbohydrates, 15% healthy protein, and 35% fat. You would undoubtedly transform the number of calories you would certainly have".

"If you are attempting to slim down, you require 600 calories less than your overall power expense. By doing this, you'll instantly obtain the additional healthy protein and carbohydrate you require to construct muscle mass, yet the percentages continue to be in place".

Applications such as "My Fitness Pal" which has macronutrient rankings, and "Fitocracy Macros" are complementary and can aid

you to reach holds with your body's demands and count your macros.

The rationale of the macro diet regimen is that you attempt various dimensions and readjust up until you discover something that matches your needs. The diet plan does not take into account alcohol.

"A glass of rosé can have around 140 calories in it - that's more than a two-finger Ki".

Macronutrient proportions

Now that we've responded to "What are macronutrients?" we need to highlight that like diet plans and health and fitness, macronutrient proportions are not one-size-fits-all. There is no excellent macronutrient proportion that matches every person, and your demands will certainly alter according to various elements in your life.

An additional factor as to why we do not advise a really detailed macronutrient proportion is that it does not state anything regarding the high quality of the nutrients. A proportion takes into account the variety of macronutrients, which implies that carbohydrates from white sugar and quinoa are assimilated similarly.

The very best you can do is:

- Focus on equilibrium.
- Focus on whole foods.
- Enjoy your portion sizes.

Attempting to reach various macronutrient targets permits you to figure out which levels function best for you. These arrays can differ, relying on which kind of diet regimen you are adhering to. Right here are some instances of macro varieties:

Conventional diet regimen macros array:

- Healthy protein: 10-35% of calories.
- Carbohydrates: 45-65% of calories.
- Fat: 20-35% of calories.
- Low-carb diet plan macros variety:
- Healthy protein: 20-30% of calories.
- Carbohydrates: 30-40% of calories.
- Fat: 30-40% of calories.

How to calculate macros and track them

Time to place our geek cap on! A calorie is a device utilized to determine the energy-producing worth of food; however, this is not one of the most precise procedures. To get a technical explanation, a calorie is specified as the quantity of warmth needed to raise the temperature of one gram of water for one level centigrade.

Each macronutrient has a various calorie degree per gram weight.

Carb = 4 calories per gram.

Healthy protein = 4 calories per gram.

Fat = 9 calories per gram.

The overall calorie net content of food depends on the quantity of carb, healthy protein, and the fat it includes. The thinking was based on the idea that if you get rid of the greater calorie per gram macronutrient, it would certainly be less complicated to minimize the quantity of food.

Chapter 4: Diet for the 3 body types (ectomorph, mesomorph and endomorph)

There are a million and one diets on the market currently. If you can dream of it, the diet probably already exists. The vegan diet is one that has been growing in popularity for a few reasons. While some turn to veganism for ethical reasons, others consider the vegan diet for environmental purposes and even health reasons. When this diet is followed correctly, there are some wonderful health benefits that happen when you begin eating healthy. Before I get ahead of myself, let's learn what the Vegan diet is in the first place!

- An ectomorph is a typical skinny guy that have a light build with small joints and lean muscle. Usually, ectomorph's have long thin limbs with stringy muscles. Shoulders tend to be thin with little width. Ecto's need a huge amount of calories and a lot of training in order to gain weight

- a mesomorph body type tends to have a medium frame: this body type is the best for bodybuilding. These body types respond the best to weight training, but they gain fat more easily than ectomorphs.

- endomorphs have a very slow metabolism and tend to gain weight, so, they should not go overboard with carbohydrates and engage in the gym. it would be better to dissociate carbohydrates from proteins.

Different Types of Vegan

To put it in layman's terms, Veganism is about adopting a lifestyle that excludes any form of animal cruelty or exploitation. This includes any purpose, whether it be for clothing or for food. For these reasons, the Vegan diet gets rid of any animal products such as dairy, eggs, and meat. With that being said, there are several different types of vegan diets. These include:

Junk-Food Vegan Diet

A Junk-Food Vegan diet consists of mock meats, vegan desserts, fries, cheese, and heavily processed vegan foods. As you will learn later in this book, our diet avoids these foods. While technically, they are "vegan," this doesn't mean that they are good for you.

The Thrive Diet

This version of the Vegan diet is based around raw foods. The individuals who choose to follow this diet eat only whole foods that are either raw or, at the very least, cooked at very low temperatures.

Raw-till-4

The Raw-till-4 diet is just as it sounds. This diet is low-fat, where raw foods are consumed until about four at night. After four, individuals can have a fully-cooked plant-based meal for their dinner.

The Starch Solution

This version is very close to the 80/10/10 diet, which you will be learning about next. The starch solution diet follows a diet that is low-fat and high-carb. This type of vegan will focus on foods such as corn, rice, and potatoes instead of fruits.

Whole-Food Vegan Diet

This is where we come in. The Whole-Food Vegan diet is based around a wide variety of whole foods such as seeds, nuts, legumes, whole grains, vegetables, and fruits. You will find that many of the delicious recipes in this book include foods from the list above. While you may think that you will be limited when you become vegan, you will need to open your mind to all of the incredible possibilities!

What to Eat

If you are just getting started with the vegan diet, the food restrictions may come across pretty daunting. Essentially, you will be limiting your food choices to plant-based foods. Luckily, there is a very long list of foods that you will be able to eat while following this diet. Below, we will go over some of the foods that you can include on your diet—so you go into your vegan journey, full of knowledge!

Vegetables and Fruits

Obviously, fruits and vegetables are going to be very high on your list. At this point in your life, you are most likely familiar with preparing some of your favorite dishes in a certain way. It should be noted that on the vegan diet, all dairy products such as buttermilk, cream, yogurt, butter, cheese, and milk are going to be eliminated. With that being said, there are some incredible alternatives such as coconut and soy. It will take a little bit of time to adjust, but you may find that you enjoy these alternatives even more—especially because they are going to be better for your health!

There will be many vegetables you can consume on the vegan diet. It will be important for you to learn how to balance your choices so you can consume all of the nutrients you need. Within this chapter, you will be provided with a list of high-protein foods—but you will also need to consume foods such as kale, broccoli, and bok choy to help with calcium levels.

Seeds, Nuts, and Legumes

As noted earlier, protein is going to be important once you remove animal products from your diet. The good news is that legumes are a wonderful plant-based and low-fat product for vegans to get their protein. You will be eating plenty of beans such as peanuts, pinto beans, split peas, black beans, lentils, and even chickpeas. There are unlimited ways to consume these foods in a number of different dishes.

You will also be eating plenty of seeds and nuts. Both foods help provide a proper amount of protein and healthy fats when consumed in moderation. It should be noted that nuts are typically high in calories, so if you are looking to lose weight while following the vegan lifestyle, you will have to limit your portions. These foods should also be consumed without salt or sweeteners for added health benefits.

Whole Grains

Another food that will be enjoyed while following a Vegan diet is whole-grains! There are a number of products you will be able to enjoy such as wild rice, rye, quinoa, oats, millet, barley, bulgur, and brown rice! You can include these foods in any meal whether it be breakfast, lunch, or dinner! It should be noted that you will need to change how you serve some of your favorite foods. You will have to say goodbye to any animal-based products and instead, try to include more vegetables and olive oil. You can still have your morning oatmeal, but you'll have to make the switch to almond or soy milk.

Vegan Food Products and Substitutions

On the modern market, you will see a number of vegan-friendly products that have been manufactured. Some of these products include vegan mayo, whipped cream, "meat" patties, and other frozen foods. While these are great to have on hand, they are still processed foods. You will want to be careful of foods that have added sugar and salts. Any excessive additives will undo the incredible benefits the vegan diet has to offer. While, of course, they are always an option, you should try your best to stick with whole foods.

Foods to Avoid

Poultry, Meat, and Seafood

Obviously, this is a given. These foods include quail, duck, goose, turkey, chicken, wild meat, organ meat, horse, veal, pork, lamb, and beef. An easy rule you can follow is that if it has a face or a mother, leave it out. You will also have to leave out any type of fish or seafood. These include lobster, crab, mussels, calamari, scallops, squid, shrimp, anchovies, and any fish.

Dairy and Eggs

Removing dairy and eggs from a diet is typically one of the hardest parts of becoming a vegan. When you are unable to put your favorite creamer into your coffee, or simply make a batch of brownies because you have to use eggs, you will begin to notice the major difference. If you wish to become vegan, you will have to find alternatives for ice cream, cream, butter, cheese, yogurt, milk, and any type of egg.

Chapter 5: The Importance of Healthy Diet and Fitness

Vegetarians Who suffer from morbid obesity and also experience Weight Loss Surgery (WLS) for treating obesity have been challenged to adhere to the weight reduction surgery high protein diet whenever they don't partake of meat, fish, poultry, or fish. The very first rule of a bariatric diet is to eat protein in an attempt to eat up to 105 g of protein every day. The equilibrium of dietary intake should be at least 60 percent protein together with another 40 percent food ingestion being low glycemic carbs and wholesome fats. These are the typical guidelines for individuals of gastric weight reduction surgeries such as gastric bypass, adjustable gastric banding (lap-band), and gastrointestinal sleeve.

To the Diet savvy, eating a high protein diet isn't any magic secret. We all know that a high protein, low carbohydrate diet arouses weight reduction. The body is made from protein. Bones, skin, bones, hair and nearly every other body are basically protein, which includes basic building blocks known as amino acids. Amino acids help the body heal from operation and gas metabolic life procedures round the clock. Together with the removal of animal proteins in the diet vegetarians have to turn to dairy and plant food to their protein requirements. Legumes, low-fat dairy foods, soybeans and soy products, and seeds and nuts are viable sources of nourishment to WLS vegetarians.

Legumes: Dried or canned legumes for example Kidney, cannellini, black beans and navy beans are supplements powerhouse foods which might be enjoyed every day. 1 7-ounce serving of legumes provides 15 g of protein. Additionally, legumes are a superb source of dietary Fiber and they're nutrient rich supplying B vitamins, magnesium, iron, magnesium and phytochemicals. Beans are flexible and may be added to salads, soups, casseroles and stir fries.

Low-fat Foods: Dairy foods are another superb source of nourishment, but patients of weight loss surgery should consume dairy with care. Some surgical procedures impact a condition of lactose intolerance in patients: it's best to check a bariatric nutritionist in case symptoms of lactose intolerance happen. When milk is tolerated WLS drinkers can enjoy a 1 cup serving of skim milk, a 6-ounce serving of low fat yogurt or some 1-ounce serving of low fat cheddar cheese every day supplying almost 10 g of protein together with calcium and vitamins A, B, and D.

Soybeans And soy products: Soybeans are protein dense: a 7-ounce serving provides 24 grams of protein in addition to magnesium, iron, vitamin B, vitamin B, and phytochemicals. However, Americans are slow to create soybeans a dietary staple, possibly due to a couple too many tofu-experiments gone bad. New soy-based products require tofu out of the odd wellness food cart into mainstream foods in the kind of veggie burgers and veggie tacos. Calcium fortified soy-dairy goods like cheese and milk are usually available in many supermarkets and create appropriate replacements for animal dairy product without flaxseed effect.

Nuts and Seeds: A tiny 1-ounce serving of nuts supplies about 5 g of protein and also a rich supply of antioxidants such as vitamin E and vitamin. Nuts are high in fat, so the percentage has to be carefully quantified. Under those circumstances, nuts can give a wholesome snack, or even a crunchy topping for desserts or salads.

Weight Reduction operation drinkers must mindfully track their dietary intake to ensure sufficient protein demands are satisfied. When protein consumption isn't fulfilled weight loss will stall or weight reduction may occur. WLS drinkers should consume a huge array of foods every day to furnish their amino acid requirements. This may be achieved by maintaining a pantry stocked with beans, whole grains, seeds and nuts and soy products, plus a fridge full of low-fat dairy.

A plant-based diet comprises a high proportion of meals sourced from plants instead of animals. This may mean eating nuts, whole grains, lentils, legumes, legumes, fruits, and veggies. However, this fashion of diet doesn't have to be strictly vegetarian. Listed below are just five of those health benefits that come from eating a Lot of plant foods:

Bodybuilding Does not entirely be based on the workout program. You also need to concentrate on choosing the proper diet which allows you to build muscle. Plant based foods play a significant role in building muscles since they supply the essential nutrition. Arranging a diet which aids in the construction of muscle isn't difficult. The meals you ought to rely on ought to have a fantastic quantity of quality protein. This can be in form of meals and also shakes.

You Should also have a correct carbohydrate amount. This aids in making the entire body to possess energy that's essential when engaging in exercises

Chapter 6: Different between animal protein and plant based protein

Perhaps you got a wise pet and determined you needed to go vegan. Perhaps you're cutting back on eating beef to enhance your ecological footprint. No matter the reason, when you lose meat into your diet, getting sufficient plant-based protein gets significant.

The Myth of the Entire Protein

To start with, it is important to be aware that it's a (quite widespread!) Fantasy Which you have to eat rice and beans together on a single plate to create complete proteins (which include all essential amino acids), such as those found in beef.

Frances Moore Lappe suggested the concept of "protein complementing" at a publication She printed from the 70s. In later versions, she adjusted the error to reflect that the prevailing scientific stance: provided that people are consuming enough calories of diverse fermented meals, they will always get all necessary amino acids and fulfill daily protein requirements. To put it Differently, rice and legumes are complementary, however you do not need to combine them together during precisely the exact same meal so as to gain from the protein every day provides by itself.

Plus, most Americans are consuming more protein than they want, so It's uncommon to become deficient (though it's much simpler without meat).

As Soon as You have Put yourself a Definite goal, write it down and Program a Listing of Actionable actions to take to achieve it. If we are adhering to the 5k instance, that may be buying new sneakers and draining out your program three times weekly to go running together with your pals. Whatever your objectives are, figuring out precisely how you are going to reach them is your first and possibly most important thing.

While it certainly is not impossible to get enough protein, zinc and B12 into your diet if you cut out all animal by products such as meat, eggs, cheese and milk, it will be a little more challenging to do so. As long as you are aware of the need to keep vegan high protein alternatives around and introduce them into your daily diet, it should all work out just fine.

Of course, one easy way to get these vitamins and minerals into your daily diet is to take a full spectrum multivitamin. There are many on the market and some are better than others. In a lot of cases, so I have been told, the liquid nutritional supplements are better than the pills because they are absorbed more easily. I don't know if that is true, talk to your doctor to make sure. Either way, introducing a quality multivitamin into your daily diet can't be a bad thing.

There are more and more vegetarian and vegan products on the market all the time. I'd bet your nearest health foods store will have a full line of vegan and vegetarian foods. Just go look around your nearest organic store and you will be amazed at your options for plant-based protein.

Along with some of the brands of organic and vegan foods you can get at your local organic store, you also have a wide variety of raw foods from which to choose. Great sources of protein are beans. All kinds of beans but especially kidney and garbanzo beans. Black beans are also loaded with protein and they can make a wild chile!

Animal-Based Ingredients

At six grams of protein and thirteen grams of fiber per thirty-five grams, chia seeds are an excellent source of protein! Chia seeds are derived from a plant that is native to Guatemala and Mexico known as the Salvia Hispanica plant. These tiny seeds also contain antioxidants, omega-3 fatty acids, magnesium, selenium, calcium, and iron! The best part is that these seeds are very versatile. While they have a bland taste alone, they absorb water fairly easy and turn into a gel-like substance. You will find later in this book; chia seeds are used in a variety of recipes from chia puddings to baked goods and even in your smoothies!

Welcome to your new favorite breakfast! Oats are a wonderful and delicious way to help get some extra protein into your diet. Half a cup of dry oats will provide you with about six grams of protein and four grams of fiber! While oats are not considered a complete protein, they have a high-quality protein, and they can be used in a number of different recipes. One of the more popular ways to include oats into your diet is to grind the oats into the flour so that you can use them for baking. Oats also include folate, phosphorus, zinc, and magnesium for added health benefits!

As a vegan, you will be saying goodbye to any dairy products. Luckily, soy milk is an excellent alternative. Soy milk is made from soybeans and is often fortified with the minerals and vitamins your body needs to thrive. On top of this, soy milk also contains seven grams of proteins per cup, vitamin B12, vitamin D, and calcium! This product can be used in a number of different baking and cooking recipes, as you will be finding out later in this book. It should be noted that B12 is not naturally occurring in soybeans, so you should try to buy a fortified variety of soy milk. With that in mind, you will also want to opt for unsweetened soy milk. This way, you will be able to keep your added sugar levels low.

Chapter 7: Breakfast

1. Peanut Butter Banana Quinoa Bowl

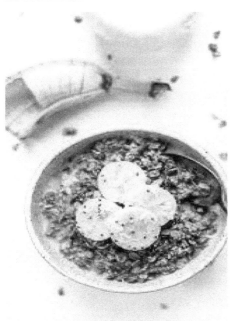

Preparation time: 15 minutes

Cooking time: 15 minutes

Servings: 1

Ingredients:

- 175ml unsweetened soy milk - 85g uncooked quinoa - ½ teaspoon Ceylon cinnamon - 10g chia seeds - 30g organic peanut butter - 30ml unsweetened almond milk - 10g raw cocoa powder - 5 drops liquid stevia - 1 small banana, peeled, sliced

Direction:

In a saucepan, bring soy milk, quinoa, and Ceylon cinnamon to a boil.

Reduce heat and simmer 15 minutes.

Remove from the heat and stir in Chia seeds. Cover the saucepan with lid and place aside for 15 minutes.

In the meantime, microwave peanut butter and almond milk for 30 seconds on high. Remove and stir until runny. Repeat the process if needed.

Stir in raw cocoa powder and Stevia.

To serve; fluff the quinoa with fork and transfer in a bowl.

Top with sliced banana.

Drizzle the quinoa with peanut butter.

Serve.

Nutrition: - Calories 718, Total Fat 29.6g - Total Carbohydrate 90.3g - Dietary Fiber 17.5g - Total Sugars 14.5g - Protein 30.4g

2. Sweet Potato slices with Fruits

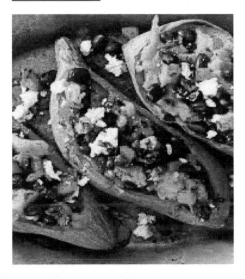

Preparation time: 10 minutes

Cooking time: 10 minutes

Servings: 2

Ingredients:

The base:

- 1 sweet potato Topping:

60g organic peanut butter

30ml pure maple syrup

4 dried apricots, sliced

30g fresh raspberries

Direction:

Peel and cut sweet potato into ½ cm thick slices.

Place the potato slices in a toaster on high for 5 minutes. Toast your sweet potatoes TWICE.

Arrange sweet potato slices onto a plate.

Spread the peanut butter over sweet potato slices.

Drizzle the maple syrup over the butter.

Top each slice with an equal amount of sliced apricots and raspberries.

Serve.

Nutrition: Calories 300, Total Fat 16.9g, Total Carbohydrate 32.1g, Dietary Fiber 6.2g, Total Sugars 17.7g, Protein 10.3g

3. Breakfast Oat Brownies

Preparation time: 10 minutes

Cooking time: 40 minutes

Servings: 10 slices (2 per serving) Ingredients:

180g old-fashioned rolled oats

80g peanut flour

30g chickpea flour

25g flax seeds meal

5g baking powder, aluminum-free

½ teaspoon baking soda

5ml vanilla paste

460ml unsweetened vanilla soy milk

80g organic applesauce

55g organic pumpkin puree

45g organic peanut butter

5ml liquid stevia extract

25g slivered almonds

Direction: Preheat oven to 180C/350F.

Line 18 cm baking pan with parchment paper, leaving overhanging sides. In a large bowl, combine oats, peanut flour, chickpea flour, flax seeds, baking powder, and baking soda. In a separate bowl, whisk together vanilla paste, soy milk, applesauce. Pumpkin puree, peanut butter, and stevia. Fold the liquid ingredients into dry ones and stir until incorporated.

Pour the batter into the prepared baking pan. Sprinkle evenly with slivered almonds.

Bake the oat brownies for 40 minutes. Remove from the oven and place aside to cool. Slice and serve.

Nutrition: Calories 309, Total Fat 15.3g, Total Carbohydrate 32.2g, Dietary Fiber 9.2g, Total Sugars 9.1g, Protein 13.7g

4.   Spinach Tofu Scramble with Sour Cream

Preparation time: 10 minutes

Cooking time: 15 minutes

Servings: 2

Ingredients:

Sour cream:

75g raw cashews, soaked overnight

30ml lemon juice

5g nutritional yeast

60ml water

1 good pinch salt

Tofu scramble:

15ml olive oil

1 small onion, diced

1 clove garlic, minced

400 firm tofu, pressed, crumbled

½ teaspoon ground cumin

½ teaspoon curry powder

½ teaspoon turmeric

2 tomatoes, diced

30g baby spinach

Salt, to taste

Direction:

Make the cashew sour cream; rinse and drain soaked cashews.

Place the cashews, lemon juice, nutritional yeast, water, and salt in a food processor.

Blend on high until smooth, for 5-6 minutes.

Transfer to a bowl and place aside.

Make the tofu scramble; heat olive oil in a skillet.

Add onion and cook 5 minutes over medium-high.

Add garlic, and cook stirring, for 1 minute.

Add crumbled tofu and stir to coat with oil.

Add the cumin, curry, and turmeric. Cook the tofu for 2 minutes.

Add the tomatoes and cook for 2 minutes.

Add spinach and cook, tossing until completely wilted, about 1 minute.

Transfer tofu scramble on the plate.

Top with a sour cream and serve.

Nutrition:

Calories 411, Total Fat 26.5g, Total Carbohydrate 23.1g, Dietary Fiber 5.9g, Total Sugars 6.3g, Protein 25g

5.   Mexican Breakfast

Preparation time: 10 minutes

Cooking time: 10 minutes

Servings: 4

Ingredients:

170g cherry tomatoes, halved

1 small red onion, chopped

25ml lime juice

50ml olive oil

1 clove garlic, minced

1 teaspoon red chili flakes

1 teaspoon ground cumin

700g can black beans* (or
cooked beans), rinsed

4 slices whole-grain bread

1 avocado, peeled, pitted

Salt, to taste

Direction:

Combine tomatoes, onion, lime juice, and 15 ml olive oil in a bowl.

Season to taste and place aside.

Heat 2 tablespoons olive oil in a skillet. Add onion and cook 4 minutes over medium-high heat.

Add garlic and cook stirring for 1 minute. Add red chili flakes and cumin. Cook for 30 seconds.

Add beans and cook tossing gently for 2 minutes.

Stir in ¾ of the tomato mixture and season to taste.

Remove from heat. Slice the avocado very thinly.

Spread the beans mixture over bread slices. Top with remaining tomato and sliced avocado.

Serve.

Nutrition: Calories 476, Total Fat 21.9g, Total Carbohydrate 52.4g, Dietary Fiber 19.5g, Total Sugars 5.3g, Protein 17.1g

6.   Cacao Lentil Muffins

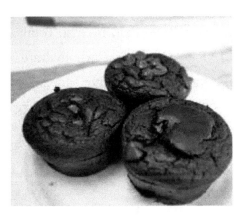

Preparation time: 10 minutes

Cooking time: 15 minutes

Servings: 12 muffins (2 per serving)

Ingredients:

195g cooked red lentils

50ml melted coconut oil

45ml pure maple syrup

60ml unsweetened almond milk

60ml water

60g raw cocoa powder

120g whole-wheat flour

20g peanut flour

10g baking powder, aluminum-free

70g Vegan chocolate chips

Direction:

Preheat oven to 200C/400F.

Line 12-hole muffin tin with paper cases.

Place the cooked red lentils in a food blender. Blend on high until smooth.

Transfer the lentils puree into a large bowl.

Stir in coconut oil, maple syrup, almond milk, and water.

In a separate bowl, whisk cocoa powder, whole-wheat flour, peanut flour, and baking powder.

Fold in liquid ingredients and stir until just combined.

Add chocolate chips and stir until incorporated.

Divide the batter among 12 paper cases.

Tap the muffin tin gently onto the kitchen counter to remove air. Bake the muffins for 15 minutes. Cool muffins on a wire rack. Serve.

Nutrition: Calories 372, Total Fat 13.5g, Total Carbohydrate 52.7g, Dietary Fiber 12.9g, Total Sugars 13g, Protein 13.7g

7. Chickpea Crepes with Mushrooms and Spinach

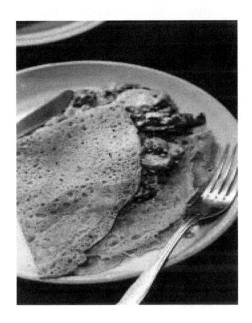

Preparation time: 20 minutes

Cooking time: 15 minutes

Servings: 4

Ingredients:

Crepes:

140g chickpea flour

30g peanut flour

5g nutritional yeast

5g curry powder

350ml water

Salt, to taste

Filling:

- 10ml olive oil - 4 portabella mushroom caps, thinly sliced - 1 onion, thinly sliced - 30g baby spinach - Salt, and pepper, to taste Vegan mayo:

60ml aquafaba

1/8 teaspoon cream of tartar

¼ teaspoon dry mustard powder

15ml lemon juice

5ml raw cider vinegar

15ml maple syrup

170ml avocado oil

Salt, to taste

Direction:

Make the mayo; combine aquafaba, cream of tartar, mustard powder. Lemon juice, cider vinegar, and maple syrup in a bowl.

Beat with a hand mixer for 30 seconds.

Set the mixer to the highest speed. Drizzle in avocado oil and beat for 10 minutes or until you have a mixture that resembles mayonnaise.

Of you want paler (in the color mayo) add more lemon juice.

Season with salt and refrigerate for 1 hour.

Make the crepes; combine chickpea flour, peanut flour, nutritional yeast, curry powder, water, and salt to taste in a food blender.

Blend until smooth.

Heat large non-stick skillet over medium-high heat. Spray the skillet with some cooking oil.

Pour ¼ cup of the batter into skillet and with a swirl motion distribute batter all over the skillet bottom.

Cook the crepe for 1 minute per side. Slide the crepe onto a plate and keep warm.

Make the filling; heat olive oil in a skillet over medium-high heat.

Add mushrooms and onion and cook for 6-8 minutes.

Add spinach and toss until wilted, for 1 minute.

Season with salt and pepper and transfer into a large bowl. Fold in prepared vegan mayo.

Spread the prepared mixture over chickpea crepes. Fold gently and serve.

Nutrition: Calories 428, Total Fat 13.3g, Total Carbohydrate 60.3g, Dietary Fiber 18.5g, Total Sugars 13.2g, Protein 22.6g

8. Goji Breakfast Bowl

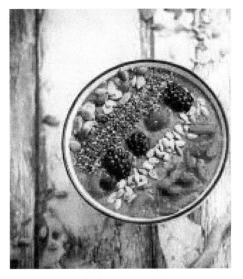

Preparation time: 10 minutes

Cooking time: 15 minutes

Servings: 2

Ingredients:

15g chia seeds

10g buckwheat

15g hemp seeds

20g Goji berries

235mml vanilla soy milk

Direction:

Combine chia, buckwheat, hemp seeds, and Goji berries in a bowl.

Heat soy milk in a saucepan until start to simmer.

Pour the milk over "cereals".

Allow the cereals to stand for 5 minutes.

Serve.

Nutrition:

Calories 339, Total Fat 14.3g, Total Carbohydrate 41.8g, Dietary Fiber 10.5g, Total Sugars 20g, Protein 13.1g

9. Breakfast Berry Parfait

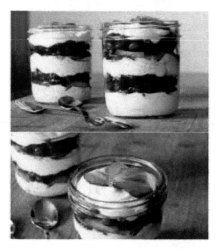

Preparation time: 10 minutes

Cooking time: 15 minutes

Servings: 1

Ingredients:

250g soy yogurt

10g wheat germ

40g raspberries

40g blackberries

30ml maple syrup

10g slivered almonds

Direction:

Pour 1/3 of soy yogurt in a parfait glass.

Top with raspberries and 1 tablespoon wheat germ.

Repeat layer with blackberries and remaining wheat germ.

Finish with soy yogurt.

Drizzle the parfait with maple syrup and sprinkle with almonds.

Serve.

Nutrition: Calories 327, Total Fat 9.4g, Total Carbohydrate 48.7g, Dietary Fiber 8.4g, Total Sugars 29.3g, Protein 15.6g

10. **Mini Tofu Frittatas**

Preparation time: 15 minutes

Cooking time: 25 minutes

Servings: 12 mini frittatas (3 per serving)

 Ingredients:

450g firm tofu, drained

115ml soy milk

5g mild curry powder

15ml olive oil

20g chopped scallions

80g corn kernels, fresh

140g cherry tomatoes, quartered

75g baby spinach

Salt and pepper, to taste

Pesto for serving:

15g fresh basil

10g walnuts

1 clove garlic, peeled

10g lemon juice

5g nutritional yeast

20ml olive oil

30ml water

Salt, to taste

Direction:

Make the frittatas; Preheat oven to 180C/350F.

Line 12-hole mini muffin pan with paper cases.

Combine tofu, soy milk, and curry powder in a food blender. Blend until smooth.

Heat olive oil in a skillet.

Add scallions and cook 3 minutes.

Add corn and tomatoes. Cook 2 minutes.

Add spinach and cook stirring for 1 minute. Season to taste.

Stir the veggies into tofu mixture.

Divide the tofu-vegetable mixture among 12 paper cases.

Bake the frittata for 25 minutes.

In the meantime, make the pesto; combine basil, walnuts, lemon juice, and nutritional yeast in a food processor.

Process until smooth.

Add olive oil and process until smooth.

Scrape down the sides and add water. Process until creamy.

To serve; remove frittatas from the oven. Cool on a wire rack.

Remove the frittatas from the muffin tin. Top each with pesto.

Serve.

Nutrition:

Calories 220, Total Fat 14.2g, Total Carbohydrate 13.5g, Dietary Fiber 4.5g, Total Sugars 4g, Protein 15g

11. Brownie Pancakes

Preparation time: 10 minutes

Cooking time: 5 minutes

Servings: 2

Ingredients:

35 g cooked black beans

30g all-purpose flour

25g peanut flour

25g raw cocoa powder

5g baking powder, aluminum free

15ml pure maple sugar

60g unsweetened soy milk

35g organic applesauce

½ teaspoon vanilla paste

10g crushed almonds

Direction:

Combine cooked black beans, all-purpose flour, peanut flour, cocoa powder, and baking powder in a bowl.

In a separate bowl, whisk maple syrup, soy milk, applesauce, and vanilla.

Fold liquid ingredients into dry and whisk until smooth. You can also toss ingredients into a food blender and blend.

Heat large non-stick skillet over medium-high heat. Spray the skillet with some cooking oil.

Pour ¼ cup of batter into skillet. Sprinkle with some almonds.

Cook the pancakes on each side for 1 ½ - 2 minutes.

Serve warm, drizzled with desired syrup.

Nutrition: Calories 339, Total Fat 9.5g, Total Carbohydrate 46.8g, Dietary Fiber 11.2g, Total Sugars 6.5g, Protein 26.5g

12. Quinoa Pancake with Apricot

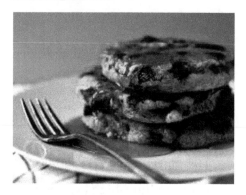

Sauce:

60g dried apricots

5ml lemon juice

15ml maple syrup

170ml water

Preparation time: 10 minutes + inactive time

Cooking time: 25 minutes

Servings: 4

Ingredients:

115ml vanilla soy milk

120g apple sauce

15ml lemon juice

5g baking soda

30ml pure maple syrup

190g quinoa flour

Direction:

Make the sauce; wash the apricots and soak in water for 1 hour.

Chop the apricots and place in a saucepan with lemon juice and maple syrup.

Cover the apricots with water and bring to a boil over medium-high heat.

Reduce heat and simmer the apricots for 12-15 minutes.

Remove from the heat and cool slightly before transfer into a food blender.

Blend the apricots until smooth. Place aside.

Make the pancakes; in a large bowl, beat soy milk, applesauce, lemon juice, and maple syrup.

Sift in quinoa flour and baking soda.

Stir until you have a smooth batter.

Heat large skillet over medium-high heat. Spray the skillet with some cooking oil.

Pour ¼ cup of the batter into skillet.

Cook the pancakes for 2 minutes per side.

Serve pancakes with apricot sauce.

Nutrition:

Calories 273, Total Fat 3g, Total Carbohydrate 51.6g, Dietary Fiber 5.2g, Total Sugars 19g, Protein 7.9g

13. Artichoke Spinach Squares

Preparation time: 10 minutes

Cooking time: 30 minutes

Servings: 8 squares, (2 per serving)

Ingredients:

340g artichoke hearts, marinated in water, drained

15ml olive oil

1 small onion, diced

1 clove garlic, minced

250g silken tofu

30ml unsweetened soy milk

40g almond meal

60g baby spinach

Salt and pepper, to taste

1/8 teaspoon dried oregano

Direction:

Preheat oven to 180C/350F.

Line 8-inch baking pan with parchment paper.

Drain artichokes and chop finely.

Heat olive oil in a skillet over medium-high heat.

Add onion and cook 4 minutes. Add garlic and cook 1 minute.

Add artichoke hearts and spinach. Cook 1 minute.

Remove from the heat and place aside to cool.

In the meantime, combine silken tofu, soy milk, salt, pepper, and oregano in a food blender.

Blend until smooth.

Stir in almond meal and artichoke mixture.

Pour the mixture into baking pan.

Bake for 25-30 minutes or until lightly browned.

Remove from the oven and cool 10 minutes.

Slice and serve.

Nutrition: Calories 183, Total Fat 10.6g

Total Carbohydrate 15.5g Dietary Fiber 6.7g

Total Sugars 3.2g, Protein 10.1g

14. **Breakfast Blini with Black Lentil Caviar**

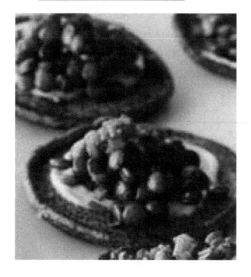

Preparation time: 15 minutes + inactive time

Cooking time: 35 minutes

Servings: 4

Ingredients:

For the blinis:

170ml unsweetened soy milk

5g instant yeast

120g buckwheat flour

75g all-purpose flour

45ml aquafaba (chickpea water)

Salt, to taste

Lentil Caviar:

15ml olive oil

1 carrot, grated

2 scallions, chopped

100g black lentils

235ml water

15ml balsamic vinegar

Salt and pepper, to taste

Direction:

Make the lentils; heat olive oil in a saucepot.

Add carrot and scallions. Cook 4 minutes over medium-high heat.

Add lentils and stir gently to coat with oil. Pour in water and bring to a boil.

Reduce heat and simmer lentils for 35 minutes or until tender.

Stir in balsamic vinegar and season to taste. Place aside.

Make the blinis; warm soy milk in a saucepan over medium heat.

In the meantime, whisk yeast with buckwheat flour, all-purpose flour, and salt to taste.

Gradually pour in warm milk until you have a smooth batter.

Beat aquafaba in a bowl until frothy. Fold the aquafaba into the batter.

Cover the batter with a clean cloth and place aside, at room temperature, for 1 hour.

Heat large skillet over medium-high heat. Coat the skillet with cooking spray.

Drop 1 tablespoon of batter into skillet. Gently distribute the batter, with a back of the spoon, just to create 2 ½ -inch circle.

Cook the blini for 1 minute per side.

Serve blinis with lentil caviar.

Garnish with some chopped coriander before serving.

Nutrition: Calories 340, Total Fat 5.9g, Total Carbohydrate 58.8g, Dietary Fiber 12.5g, Total Sugars 4.4g, Protein 14.9g

15. Orange Pumpkin Pancakes

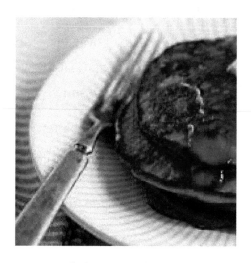

Preparation time: 10 minutes

Cooking time: 15 minutes

Servings: 4

Ingredients:

10g ground flax meal

45 ml water

235ml unsweetened soy milk

15ml lemon juice

60g buckwheat flour

60g all-purpose flour

8g baking powder, aluminum-free

2 teaspoons finely grated orange zest

25g white chia seeds

120g organic pumpkin puree (or just bake the pumpkin and puree the flesh)

30ml melted and cooled coconut oil

5ml vanilla paste

30ml pure maple syrup

Direction:

Combine ground flax meal with water in a small bowl. Place aside for 10 minutes.

Combine almond milk and cider vinegar in a medium bowl. Place aside for 5 minutes.

In a separate large bowl, combine buckwheat flour, all-purpose flour, baking powder, orange zest, and chia seeds.

Pour in almond milk, along with pumpkin puree, coconut oil, vanilla, and maple syrup.

Whisk together until you have a smooth batter.

Heat large non-stick skillet over medium-high heat. Brush the skillet gently with some coconut oil.

Pour 60ml of batter into skillet. Cook the pancake for 1 minute, or until bubbles appear on the surface.

Lift the pancake gently with a spatula and flip.

Cook 1 ½ minutes more. Slide the pancake onto a plate. Repeat with the remaining batter.

Serve warm.

Nutrition: Calories 301, Total Fat 12.6g, Total Carbohydrate 41.7g, Dietary Fiber 7.2g, Total Sugars 9.9g, Protein 8.1g

16. Overnight Chia Oats

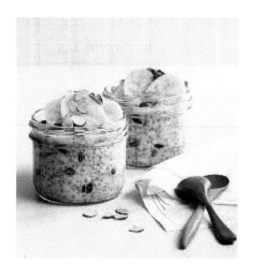

45ml pure maple syrup

30ml water

45g chia seeds

15ml lemon juice

Preparation time: 15minutes

Cooking time: 20 minutes

Servings: 4

Ingredients:

470ml full-fat soy milk

90g old-fashioned rolled oats

40g chia seeds

15ml pure maple syrup

25g crushed pistachios

Blackberry Jam:

500g blackberries

Direction:

Make the oats; in a large bowl, combine soy milk, oats, chia seeds, and maple syrup.

Cover and refrigerate overnight.

Make the jam; combine blackberries, maple syrup, and water in a saucepan. Simmer over medium heat for 10 minutes.

Add the chia seeds and simmer the blackberries for 10 minutes. Remove from heat and stir in lemon juice. Mash the blackberries with a fork and place aside to cool.

Assemble; divide the oatmeal among four serving bowls.

Top with each bowl blackberry jam.

Sprinkle with pistachios before serving.

Nutrition: Calories 362, Total Fat 13.4g, Total Carbohydrate 52.6g, Dietary Fiber 17.4g, Total Sugars 24.6g, Protein 12.4g

17. Amaranth Quinoa porridge

Preparation time: 5 minutes

Cooking time: 35 minutes

Servings: 2

Ingredients:

85g quinoa

70g amaranth

460ml water

115ml unsweetened soy milk

½ teaspoon vanilla paste

15g almond butter

30ml pure maple syrup

10g raw pumpkin seeds

10g pomegranate seeds

Direction:

Combine quinoa, amaranth, and water.

Bring to a boil over medium-high heat.

Reduce heat and simmer the grains, stirring occasionally, for 20 minutes.

Stir in milk and maple syrup.

Simmer for 6-7 minutes. Remove from the heat and stir in vanilla, and almond butter.

Allow the mixture to stand for 5 minutes.

Divide the porridge between two bowls.

Top with pumpkin seeds and pomegranate seeds.

Serve.

Nutrition: Calories 474, Total Fat 13.3g, Total Carbohydrate 73.2g, Dietary Fiber 8.9g, Total Sugars 10g, Protein 17.8g

18. Chickpea Muffin Quiche

Preparation time: 15 minutes

Cooking time: 65 minutes

Servings: 12 muffins (3 per serving)

Ingredients:

280g sweet potato, peeled, cut into ¼-inch cubes

15ml olive oil

90g chickpea flour

10g nutritional yeast

460ml water

30g spinach

40g chestnut mushrooms, sliced

35g shiitake mushrooms, chopped

Salt and pepper, to taste

Direction:

Heat oven to 200C/425F.

Grease 12-hole muffin with some oil.

Line a baking sheet with baking paper.

Toss the sweet potato cubes with olive oil, salt, and pepper, on a baking sheet.

Roast the sweet potato for 20 minutes.

Remove the sweet potatoes from the oven and place aside. Reduce oven heat to 350 F°.

In the meantime, whisk chickpea flour, nutritional yeast, and 235 ml water in a bowl. Season to taste with salt.

Bring remaining water to a simmer over medium-high heat.

Whisk in the chickpea flour mixture and reduce heat to low.

Cook the chickpea stirring
constantly flour for 6 minutes
or until thickened.

Remove from the heat and stir
in baby spinach, mushrooms,
and sweet potatoes. Divide the
mixture among muffin tin.

Place the muffin tin in the
oven. Bake the quiche muffins
for 25-30 minutes.

Remove from the oven and
cool on a wire rack.

Serve while still warm.

Nutrition: Calories 247, Total
Fat 6.1g, Total Carbohydrate
36.2g, Dietary Fiber 8.3g, Total
Sugars 2.8g, Protein 14.6g

19. Hemp Seed Banana Cereal

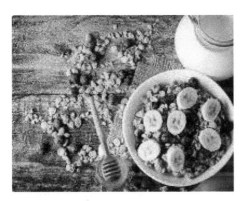

Preparation time: 10 minutes

Cooking time: 25 minutes

Servings: 4

Ingredients:

5g ground flax seeds

45ml water

70g almond meal

60g walnuts, chopped

80g hemp seeds

30g unsweetened coconut flakes

3 tablespoon coconut sugar

1 ½ tablespoons coconut oil, melted

1 teaspoon banana extract

460ml unsweetened almond milk, warmed

Direction:

In a small bowl, combine flax seeds, and water. Place aside for 10 minutes.

Preheat oven to 150C°/300F.

Line a large baking sheet with parchment paper.

Combine almond meal, walnuts, hemp seeds, coconut flakes, and coconut sugar, in a large bowl.

In a separate bowl, combine flax seeds mixture, with coconut oil, and banana extract.

Pour the flax seeds mixture into dry ingredients and stir to combine. Spread the mixture onto baking sheet.

Bake the cereals for 25 minutes, stirring 2-3 times during the baking process.

Turn off the oven and allow the cereals to cool down for 10 minutes.

Serve with warmed almond milk.

Nutrition: Calories 495, Total Fat 40.2g, Total Carbohydrate 20.4g, Dietary Fiber 5.3g, Total Sugars 9.8g, Protein 18.3g

20. Oatmeal Muffins

Preparation time: 10 minutes

Cooking time: 30 minutes

Servings: 12 muffins (2 per serving)

Ingredients:

2 ripe bananas, mashed

70g organic pumpkin puree

30ml pure maple syrup

270 quick-cooking rolled oats

5 dates, chopped

50g dried chopped apricots

15ml coconut oil

460ml unsweetened soy milk

5ml vanilla paste

12 cashew nuts

Direction:

Preheat oven to 180C/350F.

Line 12-hole muffin tin with paper cases.

Combine banana, pumpkin puree, and maple syrup in a bowl.

Stir in oats, dates, apricots. And coconut oil.

Add soy milk, vanilla, and mix until fully combined.

Divide the mixture among prepared paper cases.

Tap the muffin tin onto the kitchen counter to remove any air captured in the batter.

Top each muffin with cashew nut.

Bake the muffins for 30 minutes.

Cool on a wire rack before serving.

Nutrition: Calories 292, Total Fat 5.8g, Total Carbohydrate 52.5g, Dietary Fiber 6.9g, Total Sugars 23.7g, Protein 9g

Chapter 8: Lunch

21. Cauliflower Latke

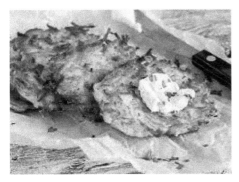

Preparation Time: 15 minutes

Cooking Time: 30 minutes

Servings: 4

Ingredients:

12 oz. cauliflower rice, cooked

1 egg, beaten

1/3 cup cornstarch

Salt and pepper to taste

¼ cup vegetable oil, divided

Chopped onion chives

Direction

Squeeze excess water from the cauliflower rice using paper towels.

Place the cauliflower rice in a bowl.

Stir in the egg and cornstarch.

Season with salt and pepper.

Pour 2 tablespoons of oil into a pan over medium heat.

Add 2 to 3 tablespoons of the cauliflower mixture into the pan.

Cook for 3 minutes per side or until golden.

Repeat until you've used up the rest of the batter.

Garnish with chopped chives.

Nutrition:

Calories: 209, Total fat: 15.2g, Saturated fat: 1.4g, Cholesterol: 47mg, Sodium: 331mg, Potassium: 21mg, Carbohydrates: 13.4g, Fiber: 1.9g, Sugar: 2g, Protein: 3.4g

22. Roasted Brussels Sprouts

Preparation Time: 30 minutes

Cooking Time: 20 minutes

Servings: 4

Ingredients:

1 lb. Brussels sprouts, sliced in half

1 shallot, chopped

1 tablespoon olive oil

Salt and pepper to taste

2 teaspoons balsamic vinegar

¼ cup pomegranate seeds

¼ cup goat cheese, crumbled

Direction:

Preheat your oven to 400 degrees F.

Coat the Brussels sprouts with oil.

Sprinkle with salt and pepper.

Transfer to a baking pan.

Roast in the oven for 20 minutes.

Drizzle with the vinegar.

Sprinkle with the seeds and cheese before serving.

Nutrition:

Calories: 117, Total fat: 5.7g, Saturated fat: 1.8g, Cholesterol: 4mg, Sodium: 216mg, Potassium: 491mg, Carbohydrates: 13.6g, Fiber: 4.8g, Sugar: 5g, Protein: 5.8g

23. Brussels Sprouts & Cranberries Salad

Preparation Time: 10 minutes

Cooking Time: 0 minute

Servings: 6

Ingredients:

3 tablespoons lemon juice

¼ cup olive oil

Salt and pepper to taste

1 lb. Brussels sprouts, sliced thinly

¼ cup dried cranberries, chopped

½ cup pecans, toasted and chopped

½ cup Parmesan cheese, shaved

Direction

Mix the lemon juice, olive oil, salt and pepper in a bowl.

Toss the Brussels sprouts, cranberries and pecans in this mixture.

Sprinkle the Parmesan cheese on top.

Nutrition: Calories 245, Total Fat 18.9 g, Saturated Fat 9 g, Cholesterol 3 mg, Sodium 350 mg, Total Carbohydrate 15.9 g, Dietary Fiber 5 g, Protein 6.4 g, Total Sugars 10 g, Potassium 20 mg

24. Potato Latke

Preparation Time: 15 minutes

Cooking Time: 10 minutes

Servings: 6

Ingredients:

3 eggs, beaten

1 onion, grated

1 ½ teaspoons baking powder

Salt and pepper to taste

2 lb. potatoes, peeled and grated

¼ cup all-purpose flour

4 tablespoons vegetable oil

Chopped onion chives

Direction

Preheat your oven to 400 degrees F.

In a bowl, beat the eggs, onion, baking powder salt and pepper.

Squeeze moisture from the shredded potatoes using paper towel.

Add potatoes to the egg mixture.

Stir in the flour.

Pour the oil into a pan over medium heat.

Cook a small amount of the batter for 3 to 4 minutes per side.

Repeat until the rest of the batter is used.

Garnish with the chives.

Nutrition: Calories: 266, Total fat: 11.6g, Saturated fat: 2g, Cholesterol: 93mg, Sodium: 360mg, Potassium: 752mg, Carbohydrates: 34.6g, Fiber: 9g, Sugar: 3g, Protein: 7.5g

25. Broccoli Rabe

Preparation Time: 15 minutes

Cooking Time: 15 minutes

Servings: 8

Ingredients:

2 oranges, sliced in half

1 lb. broccoli rabe

2 tablespoons sesame oil, toasted

Salt and pepper to taste

1 tablespoon sesame seeds, toasted

Direction

Pour the oil into a pan over medium heat.

Add the oranges and cook until caramelized.

Transfer to a plate. Put the broccoli in the pan and cook for 8 minutes. Squeeze the oranges to release juice in a bowl.

Stir in the oil, salt and pepper. Coat the broccoli rabe with the mixture. Sprinkle seeds on top.

Nutrition: Calories: 59, Total fat: 4.4g, Saturated fat: 0.6g, Sodium: 164mg, Potassium: 160mg, Carbohydrates: 4.1g, Fiber: 1.6g, Sugar: 2g, Protein: 2.2g

26. Whipped Potatoes

Preparation Time: 20 minutes

Cooking Time: 35 minutes

Servings: 10

Ingredients:

4 cups water

3 lb. potatoes, sliced into cubes

3 cloves garlic, crushed

6 tablespoons butter

2 bay leaves

10 sage leaves

½ cup Greek yogurt

¼ cup low-fat milk

Salt to taste

Direction

Boil the potatoes in water for 30 minutes or until tender.

Drain.

In a pan over medium heat, cook the garlic in butter for 1 minute.

Add the sage and cook for 5 more minutes.

Discard the garlic.

Use a fork to mash the potatoes.

Whip using an electric mixer while gradually adding the butter, yogurt, and milk.

Season with salt.

Nutrition: Calories: 169, Total fat: 7.6g, Saturated fat: 4.7g, Cholesterol: 21mg, Sodium: 251mg, Potassium: 519mg, Carbohydrates: 22.1g, Fiber: 1.5g, Sugar: 2g, Protein: 4.2g

27. Quinoa Avocado Salad

Preparation Time: 15 minutes

Cooking Time: 4 minutes

Servings: 4

Ingredients:

2 tablespoons balsamic vinegar

¼ cup cream

¼ cup buttermilk

5 tablespoons freshly squeezed lemon juice, divided

1 clove garlic, grated

2 tablespoons shallot, minced

Salt and pepper to taste

2 tablespoons avocado oil, divided

1 ¼ cups quinoa, cooked

2 heads endive, sliced

2 firm pears, sliced thinly

2 avocados, sliced

¼ cup fresh dill, chopped

Direction

Combine the vinegar, cream, milk, 1 tablespoon lemon juice, garlic, shallot, salt and pepper in a bowl.

Pour 1 tablespoon oil into a pan over medium heat.

Heat the quinoa for 4 minutes.

Transfer quinoa to a plate.

Toss the endive and pears in a mixture of remaining oil, remaining lemon juice, salt and pepper. Transfer to a plate.

Toss the avocado in the reserved dressing.

Add to the plate.

Top with the dill and quinoa.

Nutrition: Calories: 431, Total fat: 28.5g, Saturated fat: 8g, Cholesterol: 13mg, Sodium: 345mg, Potassium: 779mg, Carbohydrates:42.7g,Fiber:6G sugar3g,Protein: 6.6g

28. Roasted Sweet Potatoes

Preparation Time: 20 minutes

Cooking Time: 20 minutes

Servings: 4

Ingredients:

2 potatoes, sliced into wedges

2 tablespoons olive oil, divided

Salt and pepper to taste

1 red bell pepper, chopped

¼ cup fresh cilantro, chopped

1 garlic, minced

2 tablespoons almonds, toasted and sliced

1 tablespoon lime juice

Direction Preheat your oven to 425 degrees F.

Toss the sweet potatoes in oil and salt.

Transfer to a baking pan.

Roast for 20 minutes.

In a bowl, combine the red bell pepper, cilantro, garlic and almonds.

In another bowl, mix the lime juice, remaining oil, salt and pepper.

Drizzle this mixture over the red bell pepper mixture.

Serve sweet potatoes with the red bell pepper mixture.

Nutrition: Calories: 146, Total fat: 8.6g, Saturated fat: 1.1g, Sodium: 317mg, Potassium: 380mg, Carbohydrates: 16g, Fiber: 2.9g, Sugar: 5g,Protein:2.3g

29. Cauliflower Salad

Preparation Time: 20 minutes

Cooking Time: 15 minutes

Servings: 4

Ingredients:

8 cups cauliflower florets

5 tablespoons olive oil, divided

Salt and pepper to taste

1 cup parsley

1 clove garlic, minced

2 tablespoons lemon juice

¼ cup almonds, toasted and sliced

3 cups arugula

2 tablespoons olives, sliced

¼ cup feta, crumbled

Direction:Preheat your oven to 425 degrees F.

Toss the cauliflower in a mixture of 1 tablespoon olive oil, salt and pepper.

Place in a baking pan and roast for 15 minutes.

Put the parsley, remaining oil, garlic, lemon juice, salt and pepper in a blender.

Pulse until smooth.

Place the roasted cauliflower in a salad bowl.

Stir in the rest of the ingredients along with the parsley dressing.

Nutrition: Calories: 198, Total fat: 16.5g, Saturated fat: 3g, Cholesterol: 6mg, Sodium: 3mg, Potassium: 570mg, Carbohydrates: 10.4g, Fiber: 4.1g, Sugar: 4G, Protein: 5.4g

30. Garlic Mashed Potatoes & Turnips

Preparation Time: 20 minutes

Cooking Time: 30 minutes

Servings: 8

Ingredients:

1 head garlic

1 teaspoon olive oil

1 lb. turnips, sliced into cubes

2 lb. potatoes, sliced into cubes

½ cup almond milk

½ cup Parmesan cheese, grated

1 tablespoon fresh thyme, chopped

1 tablespoon fresh chives, chopped

2 tablespoons butter

Salt and pepper to taste

Direction

Preheat your oven to 375 degrees F.

Slice the tip off the garlic head. Drizzle with a little oil and roast in the oven for 45 minutes.

Boil the turnips and potatoes in a pot of water for 30 minutes or until tender. Add all the ingredients to a food processor along with the garlic.

Pulse until smooth.

Nutrition: Calories: 141, Total fat: 3.2g, Saturated fat: 1.5g, Cholesterol: 7mg, Sodium: 284mg, Potassium: 676mg, Carbohydrates:24.g, Fiber: 3.1g, Sugar: 4g, Protein: 4.6g

31. Green Beans with Bacon

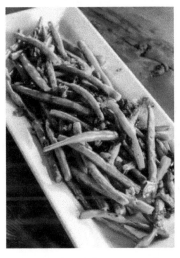

Preparation Time: 15 minutes

Cooking Time: 20 minutes

Servings: 8

Ingredients:

2 slices bacon, chopped

1 shallot, chopped

24 oz. green beans

Salt and pepper to taste

½ teaspoon smoked paprika

1 teaspoon lemon juice

2 teaspoons vinegar

Direction

Preheat your oven to 450 degrees F.

Add the bacon in the baking pan and roast for 5 minutes.

Stir in the shallot and beans.

Season with salt, pepper and paprika.

Roast for 10 minutes.

Drizzle with the lemon juice and vinegar.

Roast for another 2 minutes.

Nutrition: Calories: 49, Total fat: 1.2g, Saturated fat: 0.4g, Cholesterol: 3mg, Sodium: 192mg, Potassium: 249mg, Carbohydrates: 8.1g, Fiber: 3g, Sugar: 4g, Protein: 2.9g

32. Coconut Brussels Sprouts

Preparation Time: 15 minutes

Cooking Time: 10 minutes

Servings: 4

Ingredients:

1 lb. Brussels sprouts, trimmed and sliced in half

2 tablespoons coconut oil

¼ cup coconut water

1 tablespoon soy sauce

Direction:

In a pan over medium heat, add the coconut oil and cook the Brussels sprouts for 4 minutes.

Pour in the coconut water.

Cook for 3 minutes. Add the soy sauce and cook for another 1 minute.

Nutrition: Calories: 114, Total fat: 7.1g, Saturated fat: 5.7g

Sodium: 269mg, Potassium: 483mg, Carbohydrates: 11.1g, Fiber: 4.3g, Sugar: 3g, Protein: 4g

33. Cod Stew with Rice & Sweet Potatoes

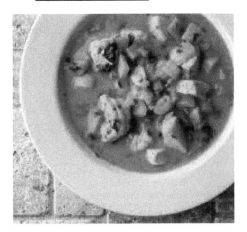

Preparation Time: 30 minutes

Cooking Time: 1 hour

Servings: 4

Ingredients:

2 cups water

¾ cup brown rice

1 tablespoon vegetable oil

1 tablespoon ginger, chopped

1 tablespoon garlic, chopped

1 sweet potato, sliced into cubes

1 bell pepper, sliced

1 tablespoon curry powder

Salt to taste

15 oz. coconut milk

4 cod fillets

2 teaspoons freshly squeezed lime juice

3 tablespoons cilantro, chopped

Direction:

Place the water and rice in a saucepan.

Bring to a boil and then simmer for 30 to 40 minutes. Set aside.

Pour the oil in a pan over medium heat.

Cook the garlic for 30 seconds.

Add the sweet potatoes and bell pepper.

Season with curry powder and salt.

Mix well. Pour in the coconut milk. Simmer for 15 minutes.

Nestle the fish into the sauce and cook for another 10 minutes.

Stir in the lime juice and cilantro.

Serve with the rice.

Nutrition: Calories: 382, Total fat: 11.3g, Saturated fat: 4.8g, Cholesterol: 45mg, Sodium: 413mg, Potassium: 736mg, Carbohydrates: 49.5g, Fiber: 5.3g, Sugar: 8g, Protein: 19.2g

34. Chicken & Rice

Preparation Time: 15 minutes

Cooking Time: 3 hours and 30 minutes

Servings: 8

Ingredients:

8 chicken thighs

Salt and pepper to taste

½ teaspoon ground coriander

2 teaspoons ground cumin

½ cup chicken broth

17 oz. brown rice, cooked

30 oz. black beans

1 tablespoon olive oil

Pinch cayenne pepper

2 cups pico de gallo

¾ cup radish, sliced thinly

2 avocados, sliced

Direction

Season the chicken with salt, pepper, coriander and cumin.

Place in a slow cooker.

Pour in the stock.

Cook on low for 3 hours and 30 minutes.

Place the chicken in a cutting board.

Shred the chicken.

Toss the chicken shreds in the cooking liquid.

Serve the rice in bowls, topped with the chicken and the rest of the ingredients.

Nutrition: Calories: 470, Total fat: 17g, Saturated fat: 3g, Sodium: 615mg, Carbohydrates: 40g, Fiber: 11g, Sugar: 1g, Protein: 40g

35. Rice Bowl with Edamame

Preparation Time: 10 minutes

Cooking Time: 3 hours and 50 minutes

Servings: 6

Ingredients:

1 tablespoon butter, melted

¾ cup brown rice (uncooked)

1 cup wild rice (uncooked)

Cooking spray

4 cups vegetable stock

8 oz. shelled edamame

1 onion, chopped

Salt to taste

½ cup dried cherries, sliced

½ cup pecans, toasted and sliced

1 tablespoon red wine vinegar

Direction:

Add the rice and butter in a slow cooker sprayed with oil.

Pour in the stock and stir in the edamame and onions.

Season with salt.

Seal the pot.

Cook on high for 3 hours and 30 minutes.

Stir in the dried cherries. Let sit for 5 minutes.

Stir in the rest of the ingredients before serving.

Nutrition: Calories: 381, Total fat: 12g 18 %, Saturated fat: 2g Sodium: 459mg, Carbohydrates: 61g, Fiber: 7g, Sugar: 13g, Protein: 12g.

36. Cheesy Broccoli & Rice

Preparation Time: 15 minutes

Cooking Time: 15 minutes

Servings: 8

Ingredients:

1 tablespoon butter

1 cup onion, chopped

8 oz. cremini mushrooms, sliced

1 tablespoon thyme, chopped

4 cloves garlic, chopped

3 cups cooked brown rice

½ cup sour cream

2 tablespoons mayonnaise

1 cup chicken broth (unsalted)

1 teaspoon Dijon mustard

Salt and pepper to taste

3 tablespoons cornstarch

3 cups broccoli florets

1 cup cheddar cheese, shredded

Direction:

Melt the butter in a pan over medium heat.

Cook the onion and mushrooms for 6 minutes.

Stir in the thyme and garlic and cook for 1 minute. Add the rice and cook while stirring for 1 minute. In a bowl, mix the sour cream, mayo, broth, mustard, salt and pepper.

Stir in the cornstarch and add the mixture to the pan.

Add the broccoli.

Cover and simmer for 6 minutes.

Sprinkle the cheese on top.

Heat until the cheese has melted.

Nutrition: Calories: 264, Total fat: 12.1g, Saturated fat: 5.4g, Cholesterol: 26mg, Sodium: 301mg, Potassium: 373mg, Carbohydrates: 31.7g, Fiber: 2.7g, Sugar: 3g, Protein: 8.2g

37. Creamy Polenta

Preparation Time: 5 minutes

Cooking Time: 45 minutes

Servings: 8

Ingredients:

1 1/3 cup cornmeal

6 cups water

Salt to taste

Direction

Mix all the ingredients in a pan over medium high heat.

Boil and then simmer for 5 minutes.

Reduce the heat to low.

Stir until creamy for 45 minutes.

Let sit before serving.

Nutrition: Calories: 74, Total fat: 0.7g, Saturated fat: 0g,

Cholesterol: 30mg, Sodium: 303mg, Potassium: 481mg, Carbohydrates: 15.67g, Fiber: 3g, Sugar: 1g, Protein: 1.6g

38. Sautéed Garlic Green Beans

Preparation Time: 10 minutes

Cooking Time: 10 minutes

Servings: 10

Ingredients:

3 lb. green beans, trim med

2 tablespoons olive oil

8 cloves garlic, crushed and minced

½ cup tomato, diced

12 oz. mushrooms

Salt and pepper to taste

Direction

Boil a pot of over.

Add the beans and cook only for 5 minutes.

Drain and remove the water. Pour oil to the pot. Cook the garlic, tomato and mushrooms for 5 minutes. Season with salt and pepper.

Nutrition: Calories: 74, Total fat: 3.1g, Saturated fat: 0.5g

Sodium: 185mg, Potassium: 438mg, Carbohydrates: 11g, Fiber: 3.6g, Sugar: 5g, Protein: 3.3g

39. Skillet Quinoa

Preparation Time: 20 minutes
Cooking Time: 25 minutes
Servings: 4

Ingredients:

1 cup sweet potato, cubed

½ cup water

1 tablespoon olive oil

1 onion, chopped

3 cloves garlic, minced

1 teaspoon ground cumin

1 teaspoon ground coriander

½ teaspoon chili powder

½ teaspoon dried oregano

15 oz. black beans, rinsed and drained

15 oz. roasted tomatoes

1 ¼ cups vegetable broth

1 cup frozen corn

1 cup quinoa (uncooked)

Salt to taste

½ cup light sour cream

½ cup fresh cilantro leaves

Direction

Add the water and sweet potato in a pan over medium heat.

Bring to a boil.

Reduce heat and cook until sweet potato is tender.

Add the oil and onion.

Cook for 3 minutes.

Stir in the garlic and spices and cook for 1 minute.

Add the rest of the ingredients except the sour cream and cilantro.

Cook for 20 minutes.

Serve with sour cream and top with the cilantro before serving.

Nutrition: Calories: 421, Total fat: 11g, Saturated fat: 3g, Sodium: 739mg, Carbohydrates: 65g, Fiber: 11g, Sugar: 9g, Protein: 16g

40. Green Beans with Balsamic Sauce

Preparation Time: 10 minutes

Cooking Time: 15 minutes

Servings: 6

Ingredients:

2 shallots, sliced

8 cups green beans, trimmed

2 tablespoons olive oil

Salt and pepper to taste

2 tablespoons balsamic vinegar

¼ cup Parmesan cheese, grated

Direction

Preheat your oven to 425 degrees F.

Line your baking with foil.

In the pan, toss the shallots and beans in oil, salt and pepper.

Roast in the oven for 15 minutes.

Drizzle with the vinegar and top with cheese.

Nutrition: Calories: 78, Total fat: 6g, Saturated fat: 1.4g, Cholesterol: 4mg, Sodium: 282mg, Potassium: 82mg, Carbohydrates: 4.2g, Fiber: 0.6g, Sugar: 2g, Protein: 1.9g

41. **Brown Rice Pilaf**

Preparation Time: 15 minutes

Cooking Time: 10 minutes

Servings: 5

Ingredients:

2 ½ cups chicken broth

½ cup wild rice

2/3 cup brown rice

2 scallions, chopped

Pepper to taste

Direction

Mix all the ingredients except the brown rice in a pot.

Bring to a boil and then simmer for 10 minutes.

Add the brown rice. Stir.

Simmer for 30 minutes.

Fluff with a fork before serving.

Nutrition: Calories: 174, Total fat: 1g, Saturated fat: 0.2g, Sodium: 265mg, Potassium: 248mg, Carbohydrates: 35.4g, Fiber: 2.6g

Chapter 9: Dinner

42. Green Curry Tofu

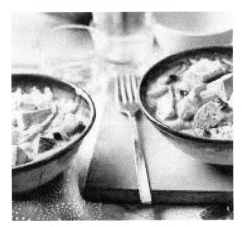

Preparation time: 10 minutes

Cooking time: 15 minutes

Servings: 1

Ingredients:

Lime Juice (1 T.)

Tamari Sauce (1 T.)

Water Chestnuts (8 Oz.)

Green Beans (1 C.)

Salt (.50 t.)

Vegetable Broth (.50 C.)

Coconut Milk (14 Oz.)

Chickpeas (1 C.)

Green Curry Paste (3 T.)

Frozen Edamame (1 C.)

Garlic Cloves (2)

Ginger (1 inch)

Olive Oil (1 t.)

Diced Onion (1)

Extra-firm Tofu (8 Oz.)

Brown Basmati Rice (1 C.)

Directions: To start, you will want to cook your rice according to the directions on the package. You can do this in a rice cooker or simply on top of the stove.

Next, you will want to prepare your tofu. You can remove the tofu from the package and set it on a plate. Once in place, set another plate on top and something heavy so you can begin to drain the tofu. Once the tofu is prepared, cut it into half inch cubes.

Next, take a medium-sized pan and place it over medium heat. As the pan heats up, go ahead and place your olive oil. When the olive oil begins to sizzle, add your onions and cook until they turn a nice translucent color. Typically, this process will take about five minutes. When your onions are ready, add in the garlic and ginger. With these in place, cook the ingredients for another two to three minutes. Once the last step is done, add in your curry paste and edamame. Cook these two ingredients until the edamame is no longer frozen.

With these ready, you will now add in the cubed tofu, chickpeas, vegetable broth, coconut milk, and the salt. When everything is in place, you will want to bring the pot to a simmer. Add in the water chestnuts and green beans next and cook for a total of five minutes. When all the ingredients are cooked through, you can remove the pan from the heat and divide your meal into bowls. For extra flavor, try stirring in tamari, lime juice, or soy sauce. This recipe is excellent served over rice or any other side dish!

Nutrition: Calories: 760, Protein: 23g, Fat: 38g, Carbs: 89g, Fibers: 9g

43. African Peanut Protein Stew

Preparation time: 10 minutes

Cooking time: 30 minutes

Servings: 4

Ingredients:

Basmati Rice (1 Package)

Roasted Peanuts (.25 C.)

Baby Spinach (2 C.)

Chickpeas (15 Oz.)

Chili Powder (1.50 t.)

Vegetable Broth (4 C.)

Natural Peanut Butter (.33 C.)

Pepper (.25 t.)

Salt (.25 t.)

Diced Tomatoes (28 Oz.)

Chopped Sweet Potato (1)

Diced Jalapeno (1)

Diced Red Pepper (1)

Sweet Onion (1)

Olive Oil (1 t.)

Directions:

First, you will want to cook your onion. You will do this by heating olive oil in a large saucepan over medium heat. Once the olive oil is sizzling, add in the onion and cook for five minutes or so. The onion will turn translucent when it is cooked through.

With the onion done, you will now add in the canned tomatoes, diced sweet potato, jalapeno, and bell peppers. Simmer all these ingredients over a medium to high heat for about five minutes. If desired, you can season these vegetables with salt and pepper.

As the vegetables cook, you will want to make your sauce. You will do this by taking a bowl and mix together one cup of vegetable broth with the peanut butter. Be sure to mix well, so there are no clumps. Once this is done, pour the sauce into the saucepan along with three more cups of vegetable broth. At this point, you will want to season the dish with cayenne and chili powder.

Next, cover your pan and reduce to a lower heat. Go ahead and allow these ingredients to simmer for about ten to twenty minutes. At the end of this time, the sweet potato should be nice and tender.

Last, you will want to add in the spinach and chickpeas. Give everything a good stir to mix. You will want to cook this dish until the spinach begins to wilt. Once again, you can add salt and pepper as needed.

Finally, serve your dish over rice, garnish with peanuts, and enjoy!

Nutrition: Calories: 440, Protein: 16g, Fat: 13g, Carbs: 69g, Fibers: 12g

44. Thai Zucchini Noodle Salad

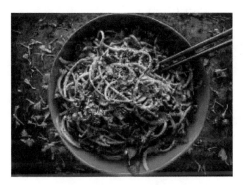

Preparation time: 10 minutes

Cooking time: 35 minutes

Servings: 4

Ingredients:

Peanuts (.50 C.)

Peanut Sauce (.50 C.)

Water (2 T.)

Extra-firm Tofu (.50 Block)

Chopped Green Onions (.25 C.)

Spiralized Carrot (1)

Spiralized Zucchini (3)

Direction:

First, you are going to want to create your peanut sauce. To do this, take a small bowl and slowly mix your peanut sauce with water. You will want to add one tablespoon at a time to achieve the thickness you desire.

Next, you will combine all the ingredients from above, minus the peanuts, into a large mixing bowl. Once everything is in place, top with the salad dressing and give everything a good toss to assure even coating.

Finally, sprinkle your peanuts on top, and your meal is done!

Nutrition: Calories: 200, Protein: 13g, Fat: 13g, Carbs: 11g, Fibers: 5g

45. Spicy Chickpea Sandwich

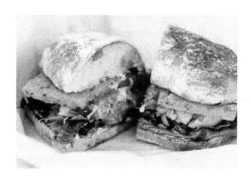

Chickpeas (14 Oz.)

Fresh Coriander (4 T.)

Salt (.25 t.)

Bread (8 Slices)

Preparation time: 10 minutes

Cooking time: 40 minutes

Servings: 4

Ingredients:

Raisins (.25 C.)

Spinach Leaves (.50 C.)

Red Onion (.50)

Red Pepper (.50)

Ground Cumin (.50 t.)

Turmeric (.25 t.)

Garam Masala Powder (1 T.)

Olive Oil (2 T.)

Garlic (1)

Direction:

To start, you will want to get out your blender. When you are set, add in the chickpeas, olive oil, juice of one lemon, and garlic clove. Blend everything together until the ingredients create a chunky paste.

With the chickpea paste made, transfer it into a bowl and mix in the cumin powder, turmeric, and the curry powder. Give everything a good stir to make sure there are no chunks in your chickpea paste.

Next, add in chopped onion and red pepper into the paste. At this point, you can also add in the chopped coriander and raisins. If you would like, feel free to season with salt and lemon juice at this point as well.

Finally, take your bread, spread the chickpea mix, top with some spinach leaves, and enjoy a nice protein packed sandwich!

Nutrition: Calories: 280, Protein: 8g, Fat: 8g, Carbs: 48g, Fibes: 8g

46.Split Pea and Cauliflower Stew

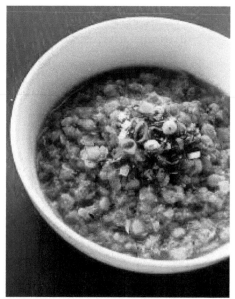

Preparation time: 10 minutes

Cooking time: 60 minutes

Servings: 4

Ingredients:

Green Onions (.25 C.)

Chopped Cilantro (.25 C.)

Salt (1.50 t.)

Garam Masala (1 t.)

Apple Cider Vinegar (2 t.)

Light Coconut Milk (15 Oz.)

Vegetable Broth (2 C.)

Ground Turmeric (1 t.)

Curry Powder (3 t.)

Minced Garlic (6)

Chopped Carrots (2)

Chopped Onion (1)

Cumin Seeds (1 t.)

Mustard Seeds (1 t.)

Spinach Leaves (3 C.)

Chopped Cauliflower (1)

Cooked Split Peas (2 C.)

Directions:

Before you begin cooking this recipe, you will want to prepare your split peas according to the directions on their package.

Once your split peas are cooked, you will want to preheat your oven to 375 degrees. Once warm, place your chopped cauliflower pieces onto a baking sheet and pop it into the oven for ten to fifteen minutes. By the end, the cauliflower should be tender and slightly brown.

Next, you will want to place a large pot on your stove and turn the heat to medium. As the pot heats up, add in the oil, cumin seeds, and mustard seeds. Within sixty seconds, the seeds will begin popping. You will want to make sure you are stirring these ingredients frequently, so they do not burn.

Now that the seeds and oil are warm, you can add in your onion, garlic, ginger, and chopped carrots. Cook these for five minutes or until the carrot and onion are nice and soft. Once they are, you can add in your turmeric and curry powder. Be sure to gently mix everything together so you can evenly coat the vegetables. After one minute of allowing the vegetables to soak up the spices, you will want to add in the coconut milk, split peas, and vegetable broth. At this point, you will want to lower the heat to low and place a cover over your pot. Allow all the ingredients to simmer for about twenty minutes. As everything cooks, be sure to stir the pot occasionally to make sure nothing sticks to the bottom.

Finally, you will want to stir in the garam masala, apple cider vinegar, and the roasted cauliflower. If needed, you can also add salt as desired. When these ingredients are in place, go ahead and allow the stew to simmer for another ten minutes or so. As a final touch, feel free to top your stew with green onions and chopped cilantro for extra flavors!

Nutrition: Calories: 700, Protein: 31g, Fat: 31g, Carbs: 84g, Fibers: 34g

47. Black Bean and Pumpkin Chili

Preparation time: 10 minutes

Cooking time: 15 minutes

Servings: 4

Ingredients:

Garbanzo Beans (1 Can)

Black Beans (1 Can)

Vegetable Stock (1 C.)

Tomatoes (1 C.)

Pumpkin Puree (1 C.)

Chopped Onion (1)

Olive Oil (1 T.)

Chili Powder (2 T.)

Cumin Powder (1 T.)

Salt (.25 t.)

Pepper (.25 t.)

Directions:

To begin, you will want to place a large pot over medium heat. At the pot warms up, place your olive oil, garlic, and chopped onion into the bottom. Allow this mixture to cook for about five minutes or until the onion is soft.

At this point, you will now want to add in the garbanzo beans, black beans, vegetable stock, canned tomatoes, and pumpkin. If you do not have any vegetable stock on hand, you can also use water.

With your ingredients in place, add in the half of the chili powder, half of the cumin, and any salt and pepper according to your own taste. Once the spices are in place, give the chili a quick taste and add more as needed.

Now, bring the pot to a boil and stir all the ingredients together to assure the spices are spread evenly throughout your dish.

Last, bring the pot to a simmer and cook everything for about twenty minutes. When the twenty minutes are done, remove the pot from the heat, and enjoy!

Nutrition: Calories: 390, Protein: 19g, Fat: 8g, Carbs: 65g, Fibers: 21g

48. Matcha Tofu Soup

Preparation time: 10 minutes

Cooking time: 55 minutes

Servings: 4

Ingredients:

Vegetable Broth (.5 0 C.)

Extra-firm Tofu (1 Package)

Light Coconut Milk (13.5 Oz.)

Kale (5 C.)

Garlic Powder (.25 t.)

Smoked Paprika (.25 t)

Ground Black Pepper (.25 t.)

Mirin (1 t.)

Soy Sauce (2 T.)

Cilantro (1 C.)

Matcha Powder (2 t.)

Vegetable Broth (4 C.)

Ground Black Pepper (.25 t.)

Cayenne Pepper (.25 t.)

Garlic (1 t.)

Minced Garlic (3)

Chopped Potato (1)

Chopped Onion (1)

Directions:

To start, you will want to place a large pot over medium heat. As the pot warms up, add a splash of vegetable broth to the bottom and begin to cook the chopped potato and onion. Typically, it will take eight to ten minutes until they are nice and soft. When the vegetables are ready, you can then add in the black pepper, cayenne pepper, ginger, and garlic. Sauté these ingredients for another minute.

When these vegetables are prepared, you can add in the kale and cook for a few more minutes. Once the kale begins to wilt, stir in the rest of the vegetable broth and bring your soup to a boil. Once boiling, reduce the heat, cover the pot, and simmer all the ingredients for thirty minutes. After fifteen minutes, remove the top so you can stir in the matcha and cilantro.

Once the thirty minutes are done, remove the pot from the heat and allow the soup to cool for a little. Once cool, place the mixture into a blender and gently stir in the coconut milk. Blend the soup on high until you reach a silky and smooth consistency for the soup.

Finally, cook your tofu according to your own preference. Be sure to chop the tofu into cubes and brown on all sides. Once cooked, place the tofu in your soup and enjoy!

Nutrition: Calories: 450, Protein: 20g, Fat: 32g, Carbs: 27g, Fibers: 7g

49. Sweet Potato Tomato Soup

Preparation time: 10 minutes

Cooking time: 15 minutes

Servings: 4

Ingredients:

Water or Vegetable Stock (1 L.)

Tomato Puree (2 T.)

Garlic (3)

Chopped Onion (1)

Red Lentils (1 C.)

Chopped Carrots (3)

Chopped Sweet Potato (1)

Salt (.25 t.)

Pepper (.25 t.)

Ginger (.50 t.)

Chili Powder (.50 t.)

Direction:

First, we are going to prepare the vegetables for this recipe. You will do this by preheating your oven to 350 degrees. While the oven heats up, you will want to peel and cut both your sweet potato and the carrots. Once they are prepared, place them on a baking sheet and drizzle them with olive oil. You can also add salt and pepper if you would like. When you are ready, place the sheet into the oven for forty minutes. By the end, the vegetables should be nice and soft.

As the sweet potato and carrots get baked in the oven, place a medium-sized pan over medium heat and begin to cook your garlic and onion. After five minutes or so, you will want to add in your cooked lentils, tomato, and the spices from the list above. By the end, the lentils should be soft.

Finally, you will add all the ingredients into a blender and blend until the soup if perfectly smooth.

Nutrition: Calories: 350, Protein: 16g, Fat: 11g, Carbs: 48g, Fibers: 19g

50. Baked Spicy Tofu Sandwich

Preparation time: 10 minutes

Cooking time: 45 minutes

Servings: 4

Ingredients:

Whole Grain Bread (8)

Maple Syrup (1 T.)

White Miso Paste (1 T.)

Tomato Paste (1 T.)

Liquid Smoke (1 Dash)

Soy Sauce (1 T.)

Cumin (1 t.)

Paprika (.50 t.)

Chipotles in Adobo Sauce (1 t.)

Vegetable Broth (1 C.)

Tofu (16 Oz.)

Tomato (1)

Chopped Red Onion (.25 C.)

Tabasco (1 Dash)

Lime (1)

Cumin (.25 t.)

Chili Powder (.25 t.)

Coriander (.25 t.)

Cilantro (.25 C.)

Avocado (1)

Ground Black Pepper (.25 t.)

Garlic (2)

Lime (.50)

Directions:

To prepare for this recipe, you will want to prep your tofu the night before. To start, you will want to press the tofu for a few hours. Once this is done, cut the tofu into eight slices and then place them in the freezer.

When you are ready, it is time to make the marinade for the tofu. To do this, take a bowl and mix together the vegetable broth, tomato paste, maple syrup, and all the spices from the list above. Be sure to stir everything together to get the spices spread through the vegetable broth. Once it is mixed, add in your thawed slices of tofu, and soak them for a few hours.

Once the tofu is marinated, heat your oven to 425 degrees. When the oven is warm, place the tofu on a baking sheet and place in the oven for twenty minutes. At the end of this time, the tofu should be nice and crispy on the top and edges.

When your tofu is cooked to your liking, layer it on your bread slices with your favorite toppings. This sandwich can be enjoyed cold or warm!

Nutrition: Calories: 390, Protein: 21g, Fat: 16g, Carbs: 49g

Fibers: 11g

51. Vegetable Stir-Fry

Preparation time: 10 minutes

Cooking time: 45 minutes

Servings: Three

Ingredients:

Zucchini (.50)

Red Bell Pepper (.50)

Broccoli (.50)

Red Cabbage (1 C.)

Brown Rice (.50 C.)

Tamari Sauce (2 T.)

Red Chili Pepper (1)

Fresh Parsley (.25 t.)

Garlic (4)

Olive Oil (2 T.)

Optional: Sesame Seeds

Directions:

To begin, you will want to cook your brown rice according to the directions that are placed on the package. Once this step is done, place the brown rice in a bowl and put it to the side.

Next, you will want to take a frying pan and place some water in the bottom. Bring the pan over medium heat and then add in your chopped vegetables. Once in place, cook the vegetables for five minutes or until they are tender.

When the vegetables are cooked through, you will then want to add in the parsley, cayenne powder, and the garlic. You will want to cook this mixture for a minute or so. Be sure you stir the ingredients so that nothing sticks to the bottom of your pan.

Now, add in the rice and tamari to your pan. You will cook this mixture for a few

more minutes or until
everything is warmed through.

For extra flavor, try adding
sesame seeds before you enjoy
your lunch! If you have any
leftovers, you can keep this
stir-fry in a sealed container for
about five days in your fridge.

Nutrition: Calories: 280,
Protein: 10g, Fat: 12g, Carbs:
38g, Fibers: 6g

52. Kale Protein Bowl

Preparation time: 10 minutes

Cooking time: 50 minutes

Servings: Two

Ingredients:

Water (.75 C.)

Maple Syrup (1 t.)

Turmeric (2 t.)

Ground Ginger (.50 t.)

Ground Ginger (.50 t.)

Coconut Aminos (2 T.)

Lime Juice (2 T.)

Tahini (.50 C.)

Hemp Seeds (.25 C.)

Tempeh (4 Oz.)

Broccoli (2 C.)

Kale (3 C.)

Minced Garlic (1)

Coconut Oil (1 T.)

Quinoa (1 C.)

Directions:

Before you put together your bowl, you will want to make your quinoa. Place your quinoa with two cups of water into a pot. Once in place, bring the pot to a boil and reduce the heat. Allow the quinoa to simmer for fifteen minutes or until all the water in the pot is gone. In the end, the quinoa will be nice and fluffy.

Once your quinoa is cooked, take a small saucepan and begin to melt the coconut oil. When the oil begins to sizzle, place your red onion, tempeh, broccoli, kale, and garlic. Cook everything together for about five minutes. By the end, the vegetables should be cooked through and tender.

Now, portion the quinoa into two to three bowls. Once in place, you can top the quinoa off with your cooked vegetables. For extra flavor,

drizzle tahini over the top and
sprinkle raw hemp seeds.
Enjoy!

<u>Nutrition:</u> Calories: 920,
Protein: 38g, Fat: 48g, Carbs:
95g, Fibers: 16g

53. Spicy Kung Pao Tofu

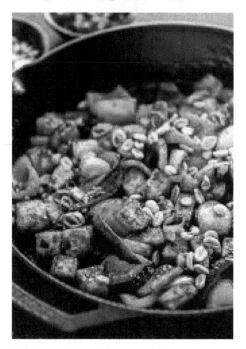

Light Soy Sauce (1 T.)

Scallions (5)

Sliced Root Ginger (1 In.)

Minced Garlic (3)

Sliced Red Pepper (1)

Sliced Green Pepper (1)

Cooking Oil (3 T.)

Extra-firm Tofu (1 Lb.)

Preparation time: 10 minutes

Cooking time: 40 minutes

Servings: 4

Ingredients:

Water (1 T.)

Sesame Oil (1 t.)

Black Vinegar (2 t.)

Cornstarch (1 t.)

Sugar (2 t.)

Dark Soy Sauce (2 t.)

Directions:

Much like with any tofu you cook, you are going to want to make sure you have pressed all the liquid out. Please take the time to press your tofu before you begin cooking, this will leave you with the best results. Once drained, you can cut your tofu into small cubes. At this point, you will also want to cut your green and red pepper into small pieces as well.

Next, you will be making the sauce. You can do this by taking a small bowl and mix the sugar, water, vinegar, cornstarch, garlic, green onion, ginger, salt, and both soy sauces. Be sure to mix everything together well to blend the flavors together.

Next, you will want to take a skillet and place it over medium heat. As the pan warms up, add in three tablespoons of your oil and then gently place the tofu cubes. You will cook the tofu until it becomes a nice golden-brown color on all sides. Once your tofu is cooked, add in the peppers and cook them for another five minutes or so. By the end, the pepper will be nice and tender.

Finally, you will gently pour in the sauce you made earlier. Be sure to stir the ingredients well, so the tofu becomes well coated. Cook this dish over medium heat for another five minutes or so to allow the sauce to begin to thicken. Mix everything well and serve over noodles or steamed rice.

Nutrition: Calories: 300, Protein: 20g, Fat: 22g, Carbs: 13g, Fibers: 5g

54. **Black Bean Meatloaf**

Preparation time: 10 minutes

Cooking time: 50 minutes

Servings: 4

Ingredients:

Chopped Red Bell Pepper (1)

Quick Oats (1.50 C.)

Black Beans (2 Cans)

Ketchup (3 T.)

Cumin (1 t.)

Liquid Aminos (1 T.)

Minced Garlic (1)

Minced Onion (1)

Chopped Carrot (1)

Black Pepper (.25 t.)

Directions:

First, you will want to heat your oven to 350 degrees. While the oven warms up, you can begin preparing your dinner.

Over medium heat place a medium sized pan and begin to sauté your onions. You can use water or oil to complete this step. As the onion turns translucent, add in your carrot pieces, pepper, and the garlic. You will want to cook these ingredients for six to eight minutes. By the end, the carrots and pepper should be nice and soft.

Next, you will want to get out a large bowl. In this bowl, carefully combine the oats, black beans, and all the seasonings from the list above. Once these are in place, add in the vegetables you just cooked and mash everything together. Combine all the ingredients well but not enough to make the mixture mushy. If the ingredients are too hard to form a "dough," add water or moist oats to help hold everything together. When your dough is ready, you can pour it into a lined loaf pan. Once in place, pop the dish into your heated oven for about thirty minutes. By the end, the edges should develop a nice, browned crust. At this point, you will want to remove the dish from the oven and allow it to cool for a bit. This meal is fantastic alone or can be served with your favorite vegetable side!

<u>Nutrition:</u> Calories: 360, Protein: 18g, Fat: 3g, Carbs: 68g, Fibers: 20g

55. Easy Vegan Tacos

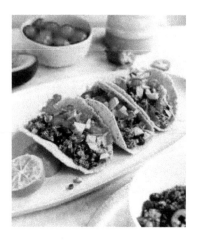

Preparation time: 10 minutes

Cooking time: 45 minutes

Servings: 2

Ingredients:

Taco Shells (8)

Corn (.25 C.)

Chopped Cherry Tomatoes (8)

Chopped Avocado (1)

Ground Cumin (2 t.)

Hot Sauce (2 t.)

Tomato Puree (1 C.)

Black Beans (2 C.)

Direction:

To begin this recipe, you will want to take a pan and place it over medium heat. As the pan begins to warm up, add in the tomato puree, black beans, hot sauce, and cumin. Cook all these ingredients together for about five minutes or until everything is warmed through. At this point, feel free to season the dish however you would like.

Next, you will begin to assemble the tacos. All you need to do is pour in as much or as little bean mixture into each taco. For extra flavor, try topping the tacos with chopped cherry tomatoes, avocado, and even corn! The options are endless when it comes to tacos!

Nutrition: Calories: 330, Protein: 18g, Fat: 33g, Carbs: 89g, Fibers: 19g

56. Lentil Burgers

Preparation time: 10 minutes

Cooking time: 15 minutes

Servings: 4

Ingredients:

Bread Crumbs (2 T.)

Crushed Walnuts (2 T.)

Soy Sauce (1 t.)

Cooked Lentils (2 C.)

Salt (.50 t.)

Cumin (.25 t.)

Nutritional Yeast (.25 C.)

Direction:

First, you will want to cook your two cups of lentils. You will want to complete this task following the directions provided on the side of the package. Once this step is complete, drain the lentils and place them into a medium-sized bowl. When the lentils are in place, gently mash them until they reach a smooth consistency. At this point, you will want to add in the bread crumbs, crushed walnuts, soy sauce, nutritional yeast, cumin, and the salt. Be sure to mix everything together and then begin to form your patties. They should be about four inches in diameter and only an inch thick. With your patties formed, you will want to heat a medium size pan over medium heat and begin to warm it. Once warm, add in oil and cook each patty for two to three minutes on each side. By the end, each side of the burger should be crisp and brown.

Finally, serve on a warm bun with your favorite vegan condiments and garnish!

Nutrition: Calories: 410, Protein: 31g, Fat: 5g, Carbs: 65g, Fibers: 33g

57. **Easy Noodle Alfredo**

Preparation time: 10 minutes

Cooking time: 56 minutes

Servings: 4

Ingredients:

Green Peas (1 C.)

Vegan Parmesan Cheese (.25 C.)

Garlic Powder (.50 t.)

Nutritional Yeast (6 T.)

Pepper (.25 t.)

Salt (.25 t.)

Unsweetened Almond Milk (2 C.)

All Purpose Flour (2 T.)

Minced Garlic (4)

Olive Oil (3 T.)

Linguini (10 Oz.)

Directions:

First things first—you will want to cook your linguini. Once this step is complete, drain the water and set the cooked pasta to the side for now.

Next, you will take a large skillet and place it over medium heat. As the pan warms up, carefully add in your garlic and olive oil. You will want to stir these to assure nothing burns to the bottom of your pan.

When you begin to smell the garlic, turn the heat down a tad. Once this is done, add in the flour and cook for about a minute in the olive oil alone. Next, you will add in the almond milk a little bit at a time. Be sure to whisk the ingredients together to help avoid forming clumps in your sauce. Go ahead and cook this sauce for another two minutes or so.

Once your sauce is done, remove from the heat and allow it to cool for a minute or so. When it is safe to handle, transfer the liquid into a blender. When it is in place, add in the garlic, nutritional yeast, vegan parmesan cheese, pepper, and salt according to your taste. Go ahead and blend the mixture on high until you create a nice smooth and creamy sauce. Feel free to adjust your seasonings as you go.

Next, you will want to return the sauce to your pan and place it over medium heat until it begins to bubble. Once the bubbles form, turn the heat to low and allow the sauce to thicken. Remember to stir your dish frequently to avoid it burning to the bottom.

As you stir the sauce, add more milk if it is too thick. If the sauce is too thin, remove some liquid and add in some extra flour. When the sauce is ready, add it to your pasta and top with cooked peas. For extra flavor, try serving your meal with extra parmesan cheese or even red pepper flakes.

Nutrition: Calories: 470, Protein: 23g, Fat: 7g, Carbs: 82g, Fibers: 10g

58. Hot Potato Curry

Preparation time: 10 minutes

Cooking time: 78 minutes

Servings: Six

Ingredients:

Coconut Milk (14 Oz.)

Peas (15 Oz)

Garbanzo Beans (15 Oz.)

Diced Tomatoes (14.5 Oz.)

Salt (2 t.)

Minced Ginger Root (1)

Garam Masala (4 t.)

Curry Powder (4 t.)

Cayenne Pepper (1.50 t.)

Ground Cumin (2 t.)

Minced Garlic (3)

Diced Yellow Onion (1)

Vegetable Oil (2 T.)

Cubed Potatoes (4)

Directions:

To start, you will want to cook your potatoes. All you need to do is bring a pot of water over high heat until the water begins to boil. When the water begins to boil, reduce the heat and place a cover over the pot. Simmer the potatoes in the water for about fifteen minutes and then drain the water.

As the potatoes are cooking, you will want to bring a large skillet over medium heat. As the pan begins to warm up, place your vegetable oil and onion. Cook the onion for five minutes or until it becomes soft. Now, add in the salt, ginger, garam masala, curry powder, cayenne pepper, cumin, and the garlic. At this point, you will want to cook all these ingredients for two or three minutes.

Once the ingredients are warmed through, add in the

cooked potatoes, peas, tomatoes, and the garbanzo beans. When these are all in place, carefully pour in the coconut milk and allow the pan to come to a simmer. Simmer this dish for five to ten minutes and then remove from heat.

This dish is delicious by itself, but feel free to serve with any of your favorite side dishes!

Nutrition:

Calories: 640, Protein: 23g, Fat: 25g, Carbs: 87g, Fibers: 22g

59. Spinach and Red Lentil Masala

Preparation time: 10 minutes

Cooking time: 35 minutes

Servings: 4

Ingredients:

Baby Spinach (2 C.)

Red Lentils (1 C.)

Coconut Milk (15 Oz.)

Salt (1 t.)

Diced Tomatoes (15 Oz.)

Coriander (.25 t.)

Garam Masala (1 t.)

Ground Cumin (1 t.)

Chili Pepper (1)

Minced Ginger (1 In.)

Minced Garlic (2)

Diced Red Onion (1)

Olive Oil (1 T.)

Directions:

To begin, place a large pot over a medium to high heat. As the pot warms up, you can add in your tablespoon of olive oil and the onion. Cook the onion for five minutes or until it becomes soft. Once it does, you can add in the coriander, garam masala, cumin, chili pepper, ginger, and the garlic. When everything is in place, cook the ingredients for an extra two to three minutes. Once the ingredients from the step above are warmed through, you will want to carefully add the tomatoes and season everything with salt according to your taste. If there are any brown bits on the bottom of the pan, be sure to scrape them up and keep stirring everything. As you continue to cook, the liquid should reduce in about five minutes. Next, pour in the coconut milk along with one cup of water. Once in place, turn the heat up to high and bring the pot to a boil. At this point, you can add in the lentils and reduce the heat back to medium or so. Now, cook the lentils for twenty-five to thirty-five minutes. By the end, the lentils should be nice and tender!

Finally, fold in your spinach and cook for an additional five minutes. Once the spinach has wilted, remove the pot from the heat and allow to cool slightly. You can serve this delicious meal over coconut rice or enjoy it by itself.

Nutrition: Calories: 490, Protein: 17g, Fat: 30g, Carbs: 44g, Fibers: 20g

60. Sweet Hawaiian Burger

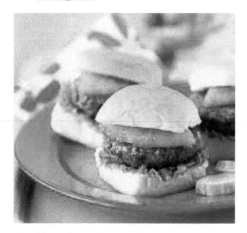

Preparation time: 10 minutes

Cooking time: 15 minutes

Servings: 4

Ingredients:

Panko Breadcrumbs (1 C.)

Red Kidney Beans (14 Oz.)

Vegetable Oil (1 T.)

Diced Sweet Potato (1.50 C.)

Minced Garlic (1)

Soy Sauce (2 T.)

Apple Cider Vinegar (3 T.)

Maple Syrup (.50 C.)

Water (.50 C.)

Tomato Paste (.50 C.)

Pineapple Rings (4)

Salt (.25 t.)

Pepper (.25 t.)

Cayenne (.10 t.)

Ground Cumin (1.50 t.)

Burger Buns (4)

Optional: Red Onion, Tomato, Lettuce, Vegan Mayo

Directions:

First, you will want to heat your oven to 400 degrees. As the oven warms up, take your sweet potato and toss it in oil. When this step is complete, place the diced sweet potato pieces in a single layer on a baking sheet. Once this is done, pop the sheet into the oven and cook for about twenty minutes. Halfway through, flip the pieces over to assure the sweet potato cooks all the way through. When this is done, remove the sheet from the oven and allow the sweet potato to cool down slightly.

Next, you will want to get out your food processor. When you are ready, add in the beans, sweet potatoes, breadcrumbs, cayenne, cumin, soy sauce, garlic, and onion pieces. Once in place, begin to pulse the ingredients together until you have a finely chopped mixture. As you do this, season the "dough" with pepper and salt as desired. Now, shape the dough into four patties.

When your patties are formed, begin to heat a large skillet over medium heat. As the pan warms up, place your oil and then grill each side of your patties. Typically, this will take five to six minutes on each side. You will know the burger is cooked through when it is browned on each side.

All you need to do now is assemble your burger! If you want, try baking the pineapple rings—three minutes on each side should do the trick! Top your burger with lettuce, tomato, and vegan mayo for some extra flavor.

Nutrition: Calories: 460, Protein: 15g, Fat: 12g, Carbs: 80g, Fibers: 6g

Chapter 10: Sauces

61. Lemon Wine Sauce

Preparation Time: 15 minutes

Cooking Time: 10 minutes

Servings: 8

Ingredients:

1 tablespoon olive oil

1 shallot, minced

3 tablespoons freshly squeezed lemon juice

¼ cup dry white wine

½ teaspoon lemon zest

1 tablespoon parsley, chopped

1 tablespoon capers, chopped

1 cup chicken broth

Salt and pepper to taste

1 tablespoon cornstarch

2 tablespoons butter

Direction:

Pour the oil into a pan over medium heat.

Cook the shallot for 1 minute.

Pour in the lemon juice and wine. Stir in the zest.

Bring to a boil.

Simmer for 3 to 5 minutes.

Add the parsley, capers and broth. Season with salt and pepper. Cook for 5 minutes.

Mix the cornstarch and water.

Stir the cornstarch mixture into the sauce. Add the butter and cook until melted.

Refrigerate for up to 3 days.

Nutrition: Calories: 46, Total fat: 3.2g, Saturated fat: 1.1g, Cholesterol: 4mg, Sodium: 116mg, Potassium: 51mg, Carbohydrates: 2.8g, Fiber: 0.1g, Sugar: 1g, Protein: 0.6g

62. **Pumpkin Sauce**

Preparation time: 5 minutes

Cooking time: 2 minutes

Servings: 6

30ml olive oil

3 cloves garlic, minced

15g cornstarch

400g pumpkin puree

300ml soy milk

45g nutritional yeast

Direction:

Heat olive oil in a saucepan.

Add garlic and cook for 2 minutes, over medium-high heat.

Add cornstarch and stir to combine. Whisk in soy milk and bring to a boil. Reduce heat and stir in the pumpkin. Simmer for 2 minutes. Stir in nutritional yeast.

Remove from heat and serve.

Nutrition: Calories 208, Total Fat 9.8g, Total Carbohydrate 20.8g, Dietary Fiber 4.7g, Total Sugars 6.7g, Protein 10.9g

63. Creamy Tofu Sauce

Preparation time: 5 minutes

Servings: 2

Ingredients:

350g silken tofu

40ml soy milk

2 clove garlic

¼ teaspoon paprika

¼ teaspoon cayenne

1 tablespoon dried parsley

1 tablespoon dried basil

Salt and pepper, to taste

Direction:

Toss all ingredients into a food blender.

Blend on high until smooth.

Serve with pasta or rice.

Nutrition: Calories 127, Total Fat 5.2g,
Total Carbohydrate 6.9g,
Dietary Fiber 0.6g, Total Sugars 3.2g, Protein 13.1g

64. Spinach Sauce

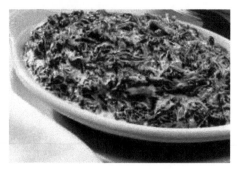

Preparation time: 5 minutes

Cooking time: 3 minutes

Servings: 2

Ingredients:

150g fresh spinach

20g fresh basil

240ml soy milk

5g nutritional yeast

15g cornstarch

2 cloves garlic

½ teaspoon onion powder

Salt and pepper, to taste

1 pinch nutmeg

Direction:

Place all ingredients in a food blender.

Blend on high until smooth.

Transfer to a saucepot.

Bring to a simmer. Cook over medium heat for 3 minutes.

Serve warm.

Nutrition: Calories 127, Total Fat 2.7g, Total Carbohydrate 19.6g, Dietary Fiber 3.2g, Total Sugars 5.3g, Protein 7.7g

65. Kidney Bean Sauce

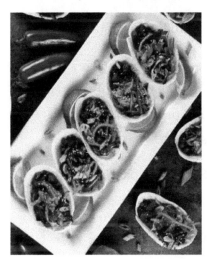

Preparation time: 5 minutes

Cooking time: 8 minutes

Servings: 2

Ingredients:

15ml olive oil

½ small onion, diced

2 cloves garlic, minced

400g can red kidney beans, rinsed, drained

30ml balsamic vinegar

30g tomato paste

½ teaspoon cayenne pepper

½ teaspoon smoked paprika

Salt, to taste

Direction:
Heat olive oil in a skillet.

Add onion and cook 5 minutes, over medium-high heat.

Add garlic and cook 2 minutes.

Toss in the beans, balsamic vinegar, tomato paste, and spices.

Cook 1 minute.

Transfer the mixture to a food blender. Blend on high until smooth.

Serve with pasta, falafel, or tacos.

Nutrition: Calories 342, Total Fat 8.2g,
Total Carbohydrate 51.2g,
Dietary Fiber 15.9g,
Total Sugars 3.3g, Protein 18.4g

66. Hemp Alfredo Sauce

Preparation time: 5 minutes

Servings: 4

Ingredients:

125g raw cashews, soaked in water for 2 hours

80g raw hemp seeds

115ml soy milk

10g nutritional yeast

15ml lemon juice

2 cloves garlic, minced

Salt, to taste

Direction:

Drain the cashews and place in a food processor.

Add the remaining ingredients and process on high until smooth.

Serve with pasta or soba noodles.

Nutrition:

Calories 319, Total Fat 23.2g, Total Carbohydrate 17g, Dietary Fiber 1.7g, Total Sugars 3.5g, Protein 13.5g

67. Vegan Cheese Sauce

Preparation time: 10 minutes

Cooking time: 15 minutes

Servings: 6

Ingredients:

450g sweet potatoes, peeled, cubed

150g grated carrots

100g raw cashews, soaked in water 2 hours, drained

65g red lentils, picked, rinsed

30g rolled oats

20g nutritional yeast

30g miso paste

15ml lemon juice

950ml water

10g garlic powder

Salt, to taste

Direction:

Combine water, potatoes, carrots, cashews, lentils, and oats in a saucepot.

Bring to a boil.

Reduce heat and simmer 15 minutes.

Strain through a fine-mesh sieve. Reserve some of the cooking liquid if you need to thin the sauce.

Transfer the cooked ingredients into a food blender. Add nutritional yeast, miso paste, lemon juice, garlic powder, and season to taste.

Blend until smooth. If needed, add some cooking liquid to thin down the sauce.

Serve with pasta, potatoes, or with poutine.

Nutrition: Calories 278, Total Fat 8.8g, Total Carbohydrate 42.6g, Dietary Fiber 9.2g, Total Sugars 3.5g, Protein 9.5g

68. Pea Cheesy Sauce

Preparation time: 5 minutes

Servings: 2

Ingredients:

160g frozen peas, defrosted

20 leaves basil

30g nutritional yeast

30ml lemon juice

45ml vegetable stock

Salt, to taste

1 clove garlic

Direction:

Combine all ingredients, except the vegetable stock in a food blender. Blend until smooth.

Gradually add in the vegetable stock, until desired consistency is reached.

Serve.

Nutrition: Calories 123, Total Fat 1.5g, Total Carbohydrate 18.5g, Dietary Fiber 8.2g, Total Sugars 4.2g, Protein 11.7g

69. **Orange & Honey Sauce**

Preparation Time: 15 minutes

Cooking Time: 15 minutes

Servings: 8

Ingredients:

1 tablespoon olive oil

¼ cup chopped shallot

¼ cup freshly squeezed orange juice

½ teaspoon orange zest

1 cup champagne

1 tablespoon honey

Salt and pepper to taste

¼ teaspoon ground coriander

1 tablespoon cornstarch

2 tablespoons dry white wine

1 tablespoon butter

Direction:

Pour the oil into a pan over medium heat.

Cook the shallot for 1 minute.

Stir in the orange juice, orange zest, champagne, honey, salt, pepper and coriander.

Bring to a boil.

Cook for 10 minutes.

In a bowl, mix the cornstarch and wine.

Add this mixture to the pan.

Stir in butter and cook until melted.

Refrigerate for up to 3 days.

Nutrition: Calories: 83, Total fat: 3.2g, Saturated fat: 1.1g, Cholesterol: 4mg, Sodium: 74mg, Potassium: 35mg, Carbohydrates: 5.5g, Fiber: 0.1g, Sugar: 3g, Protein: 0.4g

70. **Butternut Squash Sauce**

Preparation Time: 10 minutes

Cooking Time: 13 minutes

Servings: 12

Ingredients:

2 cups water

½ cup cashew, chopped

2 tablespoons olive oil

2 sweet onions, diced

2 tablespoons garlic, minced

½ teaspoon salt

¼ cup dry white wine

¾ teaspoon dried oregano

1 cup butternut squash puree

⅛ teaspoon ground nutmeg

Pepper to taste

Direction

Blend cashews and water in a food processor until smooth. Set aside.

Pour the oil into a pan over medium heat.

Cook the onion and garlic for 3 minutes.

Season with salt.

Reduce heat and cook for another 10 minutes.

Stir in the wine and oregano.

Add the squash puree, nutmeg and cashew.

Cook for 3 minutes.

Refrigerate for up to 3 days.

Nutrition: Calories: 102, Total fat: 5.3g, Saturated fat: 0.9g, Sodium: 184mg, Potassium: 216mg, Carbohydrates: 10.9g, Fiber: 2.1g, Sugar: 4g, Protein: 1.8g

71. Red Wine & Cranberry Sauce

Preparation Time: 15 minutes

Cooking Time: 10 minutes

Servings: 10

Ingredients:

1 tablespoon olive oil

1 shallot, minced

1 cup dry red wine

1 tablespoon sugar

¼ cup frozen cranberries

¼ cup dried cranberries

Salt and pepper to taste

1 teaspoon fresh sage, chopped

1 tablespoon cornstarch

1 tablespoon butter

Direction:

Pour the oil into a pan over medium heat.

Cook the shallot for 1 minute.

Add the wine, sugar, cranberries, salt, pepper and sage.

Bring to a boil.

Simmer for 10 minutes.

Mix the cornstarch and butter. Add to the sauce.

Simmer for 2 minutes.

Refrigerate for up to 3 days.

Nutrition: Calories: 79, Total fat: 2.6g, Saturated fat: 0.9g, Cholesterol: 3mg, Sodium: 61mg, Potassium: 64mg, Carbohydrates: 7.3g, Fiber: 0.4g, Sugar: 5g, Protein: 0.2g

Chapter 11: Vegan Cheese

72. **Vegan Vegetable Cheese Sauce**

Preparation Time: 10 minutes

Cooking Time: 10 minutes

Servings: 4

Ingredients:

2 pcs. small potatoes, peeled and sliced into ¼-inch pieces

1 pc. carrot, peeled and sliced into ¼-inch pieces

2 tbsp. nutritional yeast

2 tbsp. extra-virgin olive oil

Half a lemon's juice

A pinch of garlic salt and cayenne pepper powder

Minced roasted red peppers, cayenne peppers, or jalapeño (optional)

Directions:

Put the potatoes and carrots in a pot. Pour in hot water and cook under low heat.

Once the vegetables are cooked, drain the water.

Put the cooked vegetables in a blender with all the other ingredients. You can also add in the optional ingredients at this point.

Blend all the ingredients together until it's smooth.

Transfer the sauce to a serving dish. You can enjoy it with some nachos or steamed broccoli.

Nutrition: Calories: 360, Protein: 18g, Fat: 3g, Carbs: 68g, Fibers: 20g

73. Easy Nut-Free Vegan Cheese Sauce

Preparation Time: 10 minutes

Cooking Time: 50 minutes

Servings: 4

Ingredients:

340 g soft or silken tofu

¼ cup nutritional yeast

½ cup unsweetened soy milk

1 tbsp. white wine vinegar

2 tsp. Dijon mustard

1 ½ tsp. onion powder

1 tsp. salt

½ tsp. garlic powder

¼ tsp. paprika, smoked

Directions:

Combine all the ingredients in a blender. Blend until you get a smooth mixture.

Pour the mixture into a saucepan and warm the cheese over low heat. Constantly stir to avoid burning the cheese.

Put the heated mixture into a serving bowl and enjoy it with other dishes or treats.

Nutrition: Calories: 120, Protein: 8g, Fat: 3g, Carbs: 8g, Fibers: 10g

74. White Beans Vegan Cheese Sauce

Preparation Time: 10 minutes

Cooking Time: 10 minutes

Servings: 4

Ingredients:

1 cup white beans, cooked

½ cup plant-based milk of your choice

5 tbsp. nutritional yeast

½ tsp. salt

1/8 tsp. garlic powder

½ tsp apple cider or white vinegar

2 tsp. olive oil

A pinch of dried herbs and spices you prefer (optional)

Directions:

Blend all the ingredients in a blender or food processor until smooth.

Pour the pureed mixture into a pot over low heat and stir occasionally. You can add more milk if the cheese is too thick for you.

Instead of doing Step 2, you can transfer the puree into an instant pot. Set the heat to manual and let it heat up for about 5 minutes.

Transfer it to a serving dish or use it for other dishes.

Nutrition: Calories: 234, Protein: 18g, Fat: 3g, Carbs: 34g, Fibers: 20g

75. Basic Cashew + Sweet Potato Vegan Cheese Sauce

Preparation Time: 10 minutes

Cooking Time: 15 minutes

Servings: 4

Ingredients:

1 cup raw cashews, soaked for 12 hours

1 cup sweet potato, pureed

½ cup vegetable broth

1 tsp. apple cider vinegar

¼ cup nutritional yeast

½ tsp. salt

Directions:

Put all the ingredients in a blender or food processor. Blend until you get a smooth puree.

If the mixture seems too thick, add a bit more vegetable broth. Add in 1 tablespoon at a time until it reaches the consistency you desire.

Transfer the cheese to a bowl and use it as you like.

Nutrition: Calories: 236, Protein: 18g, Fat: 3g, Carbs: 68g, Fibers: 20g

76. **Simple Firm Vegan Cheese**

Preparation Time: 10 minutes

Cooking Time: 10 minutes

Servings: 4

Ingredients:

1 cup cashew or soy milk, or 1 cup water + 1/3 cup soaked cashew

1 cup sweet potato, boiled

1 tbsp. soy sauce

½ tsp. cumin

½ tsp. paprika

1 tsp. salt

2 tbsp. nutritional yeast

2 cloves of garlic or 2 tsp. garlic powder

Half a lemon's juice

2 ½ tbsp. agar-agar powder

1 cup cold water

Directions:

In a blender, combine all the ingredients except for the cold water and agar-agar powder. Blend them all until you get a smooth mixture.

Pour in the water in a small saucepan and add the agar-agar powder.

Mix the water and agar-agar powder well. Then, place the saucepan over low to medium heat.

Continue to mix until the agar-agar powder is completely dissolved. This will take about 5 minutes.

Add the agar-agar mixture in the blender. Blend it well with the pureed mixture.

Pour the mixture into your molds. You can use a ceramic bowl or silicon molds if they're available.

Place the cheese in the refrigerator for about 30 minutes or until the cheese has set.

Remove the cheese from the molds and serve.

Nutrition: Calories: 220, Protein: 10g, Fat: 2g, Carbs: 6g, Fibers: 25g

77. Easy Cashew Vegan Cheese

Preparation Time: 10 minutes

Cooking Time: 20 minutes

Servings: 4

Ingredients:

½ cup cashews, soaked in hot water for 1 hour and drained

3 tbsp. nutritional yeast

1 tbsp. cider vinegar or lemon juice

1 tbsp. maple syrup

1 ½ tsp. cornstarch

1 ½ tsp. agar-agar powder

½ tsp. salt

Half a clove of garlic

1 cup water, divided into two ½ cups

Preferred herbs and spices (optional)

Directions:

Mix all the ingredients in a blender or food processor except for the agar-agar powder and ½ cup water. Blend for about 1 minute or until you get a creamy texture.

Heat ½ cup water with agar-agar powder in a saucepan.

Add the blended mixture to the saucepan. Bring to a boil while stirring constantly.

Lightly brush your ceramic molds with oil. Then, pour the mixture into the molds.

Refrigerate the cheese for 2 hours or more.

Remove the cheese from the molds and serve.

Nutrition: Calories: 167, Protein: 14g, Fat: 4g, Carbs: 6g, Fibers: 10g

78. Vegan Nut Cheese

Preparation Time: 10 minutes

Cooking Time: 10 minutes

Servings: 4

Ingredients:

½ cup raw cashews, soaked for 3 hours and drained

1/3 cup water

1 tbsp. coconut oil

1 tsp apple cider vinegar

Half a lemon's juice

A pinch of salt

Directions:

In a blender, mix all the ingredients until smooth.

Line ramekins or other molds you have with plastic wrap.

Pour the cheese mixture into the molds.

Refrigerate for at least 2 hours or until the cheese is set. You may also freeze it if you want to speed things up.

Remove the cheese by turning the molds upside-down on a serving dish.

Remove the plastic wrap from the cheese and enjoy.

Nutrition: Calories: 360, Protein: 18g, Fat: 3g, Carbs: 68g, Fibers: 20g

79. Vegan American Cheese

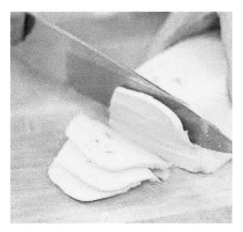

Preparation Time: 10 minutes

Cooking Time: 10 minutes

Servings: 4

Ingredients:

1 cup raw cashews, soaked and drained

¼ cup water

¼ cup lemon juice

1/3 cup nutritional yeast

1 red bell pepper, chopped

2 garlic cloves chopped

2 tbsp. red onion, chopped

1 tsp. yellow mustard

1 tsp. sea salt

½ cup cold water

4 tsp. agar-agar powder

Directions:

In a blender, mix all the ingredients except for the cold water and agar-agar powder. Leave the mixture in the blender.

In a saucepan, mix in cold water and agar-agar powder. Stir for 5 minutes over medium heat and bring it to a boil.

Once it starts to boil, adjust the heat to low and let it simmer while constantly whisking for 8 minutes.

Pour in the agar-agar mixture to the blender and process it again until everything is well-combined.

Pour the mixture into a lined rectangular baking pan that's at least ½ to an inch deep.

Only fill halfway if you're using a ½-inch deep pan (quarter-filled for an inch-deep pan).

Refrigerate the cheese for at least 2 hours or until firm.

Cut the cheese into desired sizes and wrap each piece in waxed paper.

Nutrition: Calories: 188, Protein: 18g, Fat: 3g, Carbs: 14g, Fibers: 20g

80. Vegan Cottage Cheese

Preparation Time: 10 minutes

Cooking Time: 5 minutes

Servings: 4

Ingredients:

1 ½ cups firm tofu

1/3 cups silken tofu

1 tbsp. nutritional yeast

1 tsp. lemon juice

1 tsp. apple cider vinegar

½ tsp salt

Directions:

Use a blender to combine all the ingredients except for the firm tofu. Blend until you get a smooth mixture.

Pour the tofu mixture into a medium mixing bowl.

Break the firm tofu into small pieces and place it in the tofu mixture. Mix well and serve.

Nutrition: Calories: 360, Protein: 18g, Fat: 3g, Carbs: 68g, Fibers: 20g

81. Herbs + Garlic Soft Cheese

Preparation Time: 10 minutes

Cooking Time: 20 minutes

Servings: 4

Ingredients:

2 cups cashews, soaked in cold water and refrigerated for 12 hours

Zest from 1 medium lemon

Juice from 2 medium lemons

¾ cup water

2 garlic cloves, minced (should yield 1 tbsp.)

2 tbsp. nutritional yeast

2 tbsp. olive oil

½ tsp. garlic powder

½ tsp. sea salt

2 tbsp. fresh dill, finely minced

Directions:

After soaking the cashews, drain and put them into a food processor.

Add all the other ingredients except for the fresh dill.

Start grinding and processing the ingredients until you get a smooth and creamy puree. You can taste it and add more ingredients until you get your desired flavor.

Place a colander or a mesh strainer over a mixing bowl. Then, lay down cheesecloth over the colander. Use about two layers.

Scoop the cheese and put it on the cheesecloth. Get all the corners of the cheesecloth and gather them, trapping the cheese inside. Gently twist the top to shape the cheese into a thick disc. Finally, secure it with one or two rubber bands.

Refrigerate the cheese and let it sit for about 6 to 12 hours. The longer you let it set, the better. This is to make sure that all the excess moisture is gone and that your cheese will hold its shape. Unwrap the cheesecloth once ready to serve. Place the cheese on a serving dish. You can reshape it with your hands if needed.

Coat the cheese with chopped fresh dill and add more lemon zest if preferred.

<u>Nutrition:</u> Calories: 178, Protein: 18g, Fat: 3g, Carbs: 20g, Fibers: 11g

82. Vegan Mozzarella Cheese

Preparation Time: 10 minutes

Cooking Time: 15 minutes

Servings: 4

Ingredients:

1 cup cashews, soaked in cold water and refrigerated for at least 4 hours

¼ cup unsweetened soy milk

1 ¼ cup unsweetened dairy-free yogurt

3 1/3 tbsp. tapioca starch

2 tbsp. lemon juice

2 tbsp. refined coconut oil

2 tsp. nutritional yeast

1 ½ tsp. sea salt

¼ tsp. garlic powder

2 tsp. agar-agar powder

½ cup water

Directions:

In a medium container, create a brine. Fill the container halfway with some filtered water, 5-6 pieces of ice cubes, and a few pinches of sea salt.

Drain the cashews and put it inside a food processor or blender. Also add in the milk, yogurt, tapioca starch, lemon juice, coconut oil, nutritional yeast, sea salt, and garlic powder.

Process or blend them on high for about 2 minutes or until you get a smooth mixture.

Next, add the ½ cup of the filtered water to a medium-sized pot and place it over medium heat.

When the water starts to get hot, whisk in your agar-agar powder. Whisk it well and it should start looking like gel after 3 to 4 minutes.

Once this happens, pour the blended mixture in the pot. Continuously stir using a silicone spatula to avoid your cheese from burning or sticking.

After a few minutes, the cheese will become thicker. Once it becomes thick and stretchy, remove the pan from the heat.

Use an ice cream scooper to shape the mixture into balls. Drop each ball into the brine you made earlier.

After scooping all the mixture, cover the container and put it in the refrigerator. Keep the cheese refrigerated for at least 3 hours before serving.

Nutrition: Calories: 360, Protein: 18g, Fat: 3g, Carbs: 68g, Fibers: 20g

83. Vegan Cotija Cheese

Preparation Time: 10 minutes

Cooking Time: 15 minutes

Servings: 4

Ingredients:

1 cup almonds, slivered

2 tsp. lemon juice

2 tsp. manzanilla olives brine

A few pinches of salt

Directions:

Put the almonds, salt, lemon juice, and brine in a blender or food processor.

Blend or process the ingredients until they become crumbly in texture. This should take about 4-5 minutes. Taste and add more salt if needed. Also, don't over process the mixture to avoid getting almond butter instead.

Place the mixture into about 2 sheets of cheesecloth. Use these to squeeze out all the liquid from the cheese.

Secure the cheesecloth and put it in the fridge. Keep it refrigerated for about 24 hours.

Open the cheesecloth and transfer the cheese to a container. Crumble the cheese and use as desired.

Nutrition: Calories: 278, Protein: 18g, Fat: 3g, Carbs: 68g, Fibers: 20g

84. Two-Ways Vegan Feta Cheese

Preparation Time: 10 minutes

Cooking Time: 10 minutes

Servings: 4

Ingredients:

12 oz. (350 g) tofu, extra-firm

½ cup refined coconut oil, melted

3 tbsp. lemon juice

2 tbsp. apple cider vinegar

1 tbsp. nutritional yeast

1 tsp. onion powder

½ tsp. garlic powder

¼ tsp. dill, dried

2 tsp. salt

Directions:

Put all the ingredients in a food processor. But use only a teaspoon of salt.

Process the ingredients until you get a smooth texture. Taste the mixture and add in more salt if needed. Blend it again if you decide to add more salt.

Spreadable Feta You can already serve the feta cheese after processing if you want a spreadable version of this cheese. You may also put the cheese in a container to refrigerate for a few hours. This will make the cheese a bit firmer and easier to put on a cheese board.

Firm and Crumbly Feta If you want your feta cheese to be crumbly, firm, and shaped into cubes, follow these Direction:

Line a rectangular or square-shaped baking dish with parchment paper. Use a pan where you can spread the cheese to be 1-to 2-inch thick.

Spread the cheese into your baking dish. Push down evenly, making sure that there are no air pockets.

Cover and refrigerate the cheese for about 2 hours. This will prevent the coconut oil from separating from your cheese.

While waiting for the cheese, preheat your oven to 200°C or 400 °F.

Remove the cheese from the refrigerator and take off the cover. Bake it for 35 minutes.

Take it out from your oven. Don't worry if the cheese seems bubbly and soft. It will set once it's cooled down.

Let the cheese cool and place in the fridge for at least 4 hours.

Cut the cheese into cubes or crumble before serving or using.

Nutrition: Calories: 360, Protein: 18g, Fat: 3g, Carbs: 68g, Fibers: 20g

Chapter 12: Snacks

85. **Black Bean Balls**

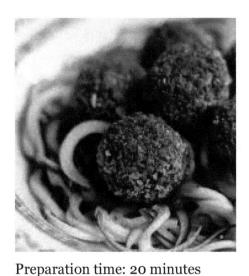

Preparation time: 20 minutes

Servings: 12 balls, 3 per serving

Ingredients:

420g can black beans, rinsed

80g raw cacao powder

30g almond butter

15ml maple syrup

Direction:

In a food processor, combine 420g black beans, 60g cacao powder, almond butter, and maple syrup.

Process until the mixture is well combined.

Shape the mixture into 12 balls.

Roll the balls through remaining cacao powder.

Place the balls in a refrigerator for 10 minutes.

Serve.

Nutrition:

Calories 245, Total Fat 3g, Total Carbohydrate 41.4g, Dietary Fiber 17.1g, Total Sugars 3.1g, Protein 13.1g

86. Chickpea Choco Slices

Preparation time: 10 minutes

Cooking time: 50 minutes

Servings: 12 slices, 2 per serving

Ingredients:

400g can chickpeas, rinsed, drained

250g almond butter

70ml maple syrup

15ml vanilla paste

1 pinch salt

2g baking powder

2g baking soda

40g vegan chocolate chips

Direction:

Preheat oven to 180C/350F.

Grease large baking pan with coconut oil.

Combine chickpeas, almond butter, maple syrup, vanilla, salt, baking powder, and baking soda in a food blender.

Blend until smooth. Stir in half the chocolate chips-

Spread the batter into the prepared baking pan.

Sprinkle with reserved chocolate chips.

Bake for 45-50 minutes or until an inserted toothpick comes out clean.

Cool on a wire rack for 20 minutes. slice and serve.

Nutrition: Calories 426, Total Fat 27.2g, Total Carbohydrate 39.2g, Dietary Fiber 4.9g, Total Sugars 15.7g, Protein 10g

87. Sweet Green Cookies

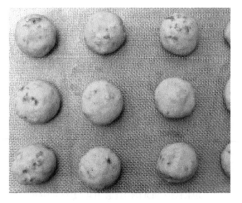

Preparation time: 10 minutes

Cooking time: 30 minutes

Servings: 12 cookies, 3 per serving

Ingredients:

165g green peas

80g chopped Medjool dates

60g silken tofu, mashed

100g almond flour

1 teaspoon baking powder

12 almonds

Direction:

Preheat oven to 180C/350F.

Combine peas and dates in a food processor.

Process until the thick paste is formed.

Transfer the pea mixture into a bowl. Stir in tofu, almond flour, and baking powder.

Shape the mixture into 12 balls.

Arrange balls onto baking sheet, lined with parchment paper. Flatten each ball with oiled palm.

Insert an almond into each cookie. Bake the cookies for 25-30 minutes or until gently golden.

Cool on a wire rack before serving.

Nutrition: Calories 221, Total Fat 10.3g, Total Carbohydrate 26.2g, Dietary Fiber 6g, Total Sugars 15.1g, Protein 8.2g

88. Chickpea Cookie Dough

Preparation time: 10 minutes

Servings: 4

Ingredients:

400g can chickpeas, rinsed, drained

130g smooth peanut butter

10ml vanilla extract

½ teaspoon cinnamon

10g chia seeds

40g quality dark Vegan chocolate chips

Direction:

Drain chickpeas in a colander. Remove the skin from the chickpeas. Place chickpeas, peanut butter, vanilla, cinnamon, and chia in a food blender. Blend until smooth.

Stir in chocolate chips and divide among four serving bowls.

Serve.

Nutrition: Calories 376, Total Fat 20.9g, Total Carbohydrate 37.2g, Dietary Fiber 7.3g, Total Sugars 3.3g, Protein 14.2g

89. **Banana Bars**

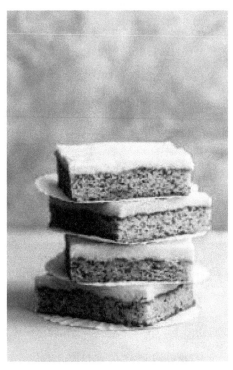

95g cooked quinoa

25g chia seeds

5ml vanilla

90g quick cooking oats

55g whole-wheat flour

5g baking powder

5g cinnamon

1 pinch salt

Topping:

5ml melted coconut oil

30g vegan chocolate, chopped

Preparation time: 10 minutes

Cooking time: 30 minutes

Servings: 8

Ingredients:

130g smooth peanut butter

60ml maple syrup

1 banana, mashed

45ml water

15g ground flax seeds

Direction:

Preheat oven to 180C/350F.

Line 16cm baking dish with parchment paper.

Combine flax seeds and water in a small bowl. Place aside 10 minutes.

In a separate bowl, combine peanut butter, maple syrup, and banana. Fold in the flax seeds mixture.

Once you have a smooth mixture, stir in quinoa, chia seeds, vanilla extract, oat, whole-wheat flour, baking powder, cinnamon, and salt.

Pour the batter into prepared baking dish. Cut into 8 bars.

Bake the bars for 30 minutes.

In the meantime, make the topping; combine chocolate and coconut oil in a heatproof bowl. Set over simmering water, until melted.

Remove the bars from the oven. Place on a wire rack for 15 minutes to cool.

Remove the bars from the baking dish, and drizzle with chocolate topping.

Serve.

Nutrition:

Calories 278, Total Fat 11.9g, Total Carbohydrate 35.5g, Dietary Fiber 5.8g, Total Sugars 10.8g, Protein 9.4g

90. Protein Donuts

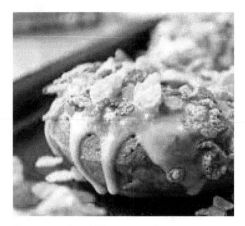

Preparation Time: 5 minutes

Cooking Time: 20 minutes

Servings: 10 donuts, 2 per serving

Ingredients:

85g coconut flour

110g vanilla flavored germinated brown rice protein powder

25g almond flour

50g maple sugar

30ml melted coconut oil

8g baking powder

115ml soy milk

½ teaspoon apple cider vinegar

½ teaspoon vanilla paste

½ teaspoon cinnamon

30ml organic applesauce

Additional:

30g powdered coconut sugar

10g cinnamon

Directions:

In a bowl, combine all the dry ingredients.

In a separate bowl, whisk the milk with applesauce, coconut oil, and cider vinegar.

Fold the wet ingredients into dry and stir until blended thoroughly.

Heat oven to 180C/350F and grease 10-hole donut pan.

Spoon the prepared batter into greased donut pan.

Bake the donuts for 15-20 minutes.

While the donuts are still warm, sprinkle with coconut sugar and cinnamon.

Serve warm.

<u>Nutrition:</u> Calories 270, Total Fat 9.3g, Total Carbohydrate 28.4g, Dietary Fiber 10.2g, Total Sugars 10.1g, Protein 20.5g

91. <u>**Lentil Balls**</u>

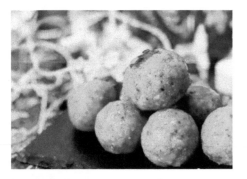

Preparation time: 10 minutes

Servings: 16 balls, 2 per serving

Ingredients:

150g cooked green lentils

10ml coconut oil

5g coconut sugar

180g quick cooking oats

40g unsweetened coconut, shredded

40g raw pumpkin seeds

110g peanut butter

40ml maple syrup

Direction:

Combine all ingredients in a large bowl, as listed.

Shape the mixture into 16 balls.

Arrange the balls onto a plate, lined with parchment paper.

Refrigerate 30 minutes.

Serve.

<u>Nutrition:</u> Calories 305, Total Fat 13.7g, Total Carbohydrate 35.4g, Dietary Fiber 9.5g, Total Sugars 6.3g, Protein 12.6g

92. Homemade granola

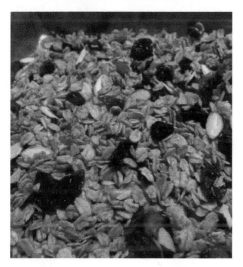

Preparation time: 10 minutes

Cooking time: 24 minutes

Servings: 8

Ingredients:

270g rolled oats

100g coconut flakes

40g pumpkin seeds

80g hemp seeds

30ml coconut oil

70ml maple syrup

50g Goji berries

Direction:

Combine all ingredients on a large baking sheet.

Preheat oven to 180C°/350F.

Bake the granola for 12 minutes. Remove from the oven and stir.

Bake an additional 12 minutes.

Serve at room temperature.

Nutrition: Calories 344, Total Fat 17.4g, Total Carbohydrate 39.7g, Dietary Fiber 5.8g, Total Sugars 12.9g, Protein 9.9g

93. Cookie Almond Balls

Preparation time: 15 minutes

Servings: 16 balls, 2 per serving

Ingredients:

100g almond meal

60g vanilla flavored rice protein powder

80g almond butter or any nut butter

10 drops Stevia

15ml coconut oil

15g coconut cream

40g vegan chocolate chips

Direction:

Combine almond meal and protein powder in a large bowl.

Fold in almond butter, Stevia, coconut oil, and coconut cream.

If the mixture is too crumbly, add some water. Fold in chopped chocolate and stir until combined.

Shape the mixture into 16 balls.

You can additionally roll the balls into almond flour.

Serve.

Nutrition: Calories 132, Total Fat 8.4g,
Total Carbohydrate 6.7g, Dietary Fiber 2.2g, Total Sugars 3.1g, Protein 8.1g

94. Spiced Dutch Cookies

Preparation time: 20 minutes

Cooking time: 8 minutes

Servings: 6

Ingredients:

180g almond flour

55ml coconut oil, melted

60g rice protein powder, vanilla flavor

1 banana, mashed

40g Chia seeds

Spice mix:

15g allspice

1 pinch white pepper

1 pinch ground coriander seeds

1 pinch ground mace

Direction:

Preheat oven to 190C/375F.

Soak chia seeds in ½ cup water. Place aside 10 minutes.

Mash banana in a large bowl. Fold in almond flour, coconut oil, protein powder, and spice mix.

Add soaked chia seeds and stir to combine.

Stir until the dough is combined and soft. If needed add 1-2 tablespoons water. Roll the dough to 1cm thick. Cut out cookies. Arrange the cookies onto baking

sheet lined with parchment paper. Bake 7-8 minutes.

Serve at room temperature.

Nutrition: Calories 278, Total Fat 20g, Total Carbohydrate 13.1g, Dietary Fiber 5.9g, Total Sugars 2.4g,
Protein 13.1

Chapter 13: Shopping list

-soy milk

-chia seeds

-Peanut Sauce

-Green Onions

-Zucchini

-wild rice

-edamame

-Salt

-pecans

-cashew or soy milk

-soy sauce

-paprika

-lemons

-Brussels sprouts

-soy sauce

-Carrots

-Pepper

- rolled oats

-butter

-Extra-firm Tofu

-Carrot   -

-brown rice

-vegetable stock

-onions

-dried cherries

-red wine vinegar

-sweet potato

-cumin

-garlic

-maple syrup

-coconut oil

-Red Lentils

-Sweet Potato

-Ginger

-Chili Powder   -curry powder

-olive oil   -scallions

-corn kernels   -cherry tomatoes

-baby spinach   -fresh basil

-walnuts   -pistachios

--Blackberry Jam   -coconut flour

-vanilla flavored germinated brown rice protein powder

-almond flour   -maple sugar

-melted coconut oil   -baking powder

-soy milk   -apple cider vinegar

-vanilla paste   -cinnamon

-organic applesauce   -blackberries

-pure maple syrup   -chia seeds

Chapter 14: 24 Days High Protein Meal Plan

DAYS	BREAKFAST	LUNCH/DINNER	SNACKS/VEGAN CHEESE
1	Peanut Butter Banana Quinoa Bowl	Cauliflower Latke	Vegan Vegetable Cheese Sauce
2	Orange Pumpkin Pancakes	Roasted Brussels Sprouts	Easy Nut-Free Vegan Cheese Sauce
3	Sweet Potato slices with Fruits	Brussels Sprouts & Cranberries Salad	White Beans Vegan Cheese Sauce
4	Breakfast Oat Brownies	Potato Latke	Basic Cashew + Sweet Potato Vegan Cheese Sauce
5	Spinach Tofu Scramble with Sour Cream	Broccoli Rabe	Simple Firm Vegan Cheese
6	Overnight Chia Oats	Whipped Potatoes	Easy Cashew Vegan Cheese
7	Mexican Breakfast	Quinoa Avocado Salad	Vegan Nut Cheese

8	Amaranth Quinoa porridge	Roasted Sweet Potatoes	Vegan American Cheese
9	Cacao Lentil Muffins	Cauliflower Salad	Vegan Cottage Cheese
10	Chickpea Crepes with Mushrooms and Spinach	Garlic Mashed Potatoes & Turnips	Herbs + Garlic Soft Cheese
11	Goji Breakfast Bowl	Green Beans with Bacon	Vegan Mozzarella Cheese
12	Breakfast Berry Parfait	Coconut Brussels Sprouts	Vegan Cotija Cheese
13	Mini Tofu Frittatas	Cod Stew with Rice & Sweet Potatoes	Two-Ways Vegan Feta Cheese
14	Brownie Pancakes	Chicken & Rice	Black Bean Balls
15	Chickpea Muffin Quiche	Rice Bowl with Edamame	Chickpea Choco Slices
16	Quinoa Pancake with Apricot	Cheesy Broccoli & Rice	Sweet Green Cookies

17	Artichoke Spinach Squares	Creamy Polenta	Chickpea Cookie Dough
18	Breakfast Blini with Black Lentil Caviar	Skillet Quinoa	Banana Bars
19	Hemp Seed Banana Cereal	Green Beans with Balsamic Sauce	Protein Donuts
20	Oatmeal Muffins	Sautéed Garlic Green Beans	Lentil Balls
21	Peanut Butter Banana Quinoa Bowl	Brown Rice Pilaf	Homemade granola
22	Orange Pumpkin Pancakes	Green Curry Tofu	Cookie Almond Balls
23	Sweet Potato slices with Fruits	African Peanut Protein Stew	Spiced Dutch Cookies
24	Breakfast Oat Brownies	Thai Zucchini Noodle Salad	Black Bean Balls

Conclusion

I would like to thank you once again for downloading my book, and I hope you enjoyed it. Hopefully, I was able to clarify why it is so important that we have protein in our diet and how you CAN do it as a vegan.

So, do not be afraid of this diet and feel that you are not capable of reaching the lifestyle that you desire! Yes, it may take time but do not be scared to make the transition. With a little effort, research and dedication, you will find that it is much easier to live a healthy vegan lifestyle! Happy reading!

There are going to be many doubters out there in the world—do not let them convince you that your diet is wrong. You are the only person you need to convince that a vegan diet is the best option for you. You have made the decision to not only better your health but also make the world around you better. At this point, you are saving animals and helping the environment. Your diet choices are beneficial to you and the world around you. Now, you know just how delicious your diet can be. While some look at a vegan diet as restrictive, you know better. As a vegan, you get to have your cake and eat it as well!   Best of luck to you and I hope this book helps you make amazing tasting vegan recipes.

CPSIA information can be obtained
at www.ICGtesting.com
Printed in the USA
LVHW080401290321
682800LV00002B/21